The pathology of deafness

An introduction

Mary Ingle Wright

M R C S L R C P D C P (Lond) M R C Path Ph D (Lond)

Senior Lecturer in Otolaryngology
University of Manchester

formerly Senior Lecturer in Clinical Pathology
Institute of Laryngology and Otology
University of London

Manchester University Press
The Williams & Wilkins Company

Published by the University of Manchester at
THE UNIVERSITY PRESS
316–324 Oxford Road, Manchester M13 9NR

ISBN 0 7190 0418 7

Distributed in the USA by
THE WILLIAMS & WILKINS COMPANY
428 East Preston Street, Baltimore, Md 21202

Made and printed in Great Britain by
William Clowes & Sons, Limited
London, Beccles and Colchester

The pathology of deafness

Contents

Illustrations

Foreword

Even in an age which realises the dangers of one branch of knowledge developing in isolation from those properly germane to it, the scientific study of the causes of deafness probably exemplifies isolation more than any other branch of medicine. Unlike the eye, the ear is often regarded by physicians as irrelevant to their study of the whole patient. This leads inevitably to some obscurity in the literature of the pathology of the deafness associated with some general diseases. This small book, which is little more than a list of references that I have found useful, was written to help me understand the literature from a pathologist's point of view. I hope it may be of some interest to physicians and paediatricians as well as to otologists and pathologists.

It is a pleasure to acknowledge the help of many colleagues, including Dr R. W. Smithells, now Professor of Paediatrics in the University of Leeds, for permission to reproduce the punch card in use at the Liverpool Congenital Malformations Registry, and the Midwifery Superintendent at Guy's Hospital for the details of the 'at risk' register. I am grateful for useful discussion and information on prospective surveys of pregnancies complicated by virus infection to Dr Bruce White and Professor J. C. McDonald. All my former colleagues at the Institute of Laryngology and Otology helped me, but in particular I am grateful to Professor I. Friedmann for his continuing interest.

M. I. W.

The problems of deafness are deeper and more complex, if not more important, than those of blindness. Deafness is a much worse misfortune. For it means loss of the most vital stimulus—the sound of the voice—that brings language, sets thoughts astir, and keeps us in the intellectual company of man.

Helen Keller in a letter to J. Kerr Love
in *The Deaf Child* by J. Kerr Love, London, Simpkin & Co., 1911

The ears have not attracted sufficient attention from pathologists, who, with few exceptions, have fought shy of the apparently barren regions of the temporal bone.

I. Friedmann in *Systemic Pathology*, vol. II, p. 1651,
ed. G. Payling Wright and W. St C. Symmers, London, Longmans Green & Co., 1966

I Introduction

It is difficult not to define pathology so broadly that it includes the whole of medicine. Whatever the original use of the word, it has now come to mean the scientific study of disease, with particular reference to causes and the characteristic microscopical appearances of cellular activity.

Causes must include chromosomal aberrations, for many of which no ultimate cause has yet been found, and inherited defects, as well as the results of infection, degeneration, poisoning of tissues, trauma, and neoplasia.

Physiological defect due to remote pathology, such as absence of action of an essential hormone, is perhaps less obviously part of pathology. Yet where a condition is associated with a known lack of a certain hormone it is important not to omit it entirely from consideration. Advances in knowledge of cellular enzymes and biochemical processes elsewhere in the body may precede such knowledge in a particular field and yet be relevant to it. To some extent the pathologist must be aware of such possibilities if the best use is to be made of clinical material for the advancement of knowledge.

All these fields are involved in the pathology of hearing loss, which nearly always arises from disease of the middle ear, cochlea or statoacoustic nerve.

In a comprehensive review article on profound childhood deafness Fraser (1964) underlines the impossibility of an unambiguous classification of deafness, because congenital and post-natal deafness cannot be wholly equated with genetic and acquired forms. Nor is the term 'profound childhood deafness', in itself a socio-educational entity, comprehensive of all forms of deafness. It excludes those genetical syndromes which appear in later life, and also those in which the deafness plays a minor part.

Fraser classifies deafness initially as in table 1.

Table I

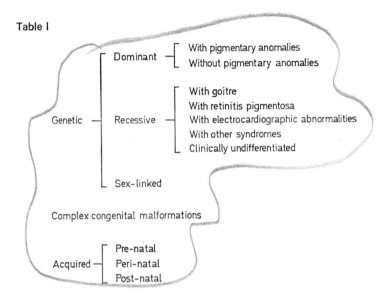

Genetic
  Dominant
    With pigmentary anomalies
    Without pigmentary anomalies
  Recessive
    With goitre
    With retinitis pigmentosa
    With electrocardiographic abnormalities
    With other syndromes
    Clinically undifferentiated
  Sex-linked

Complex congenital malformations

Acquired
  Pre-natal
  Peri-natal
  Post-natal

A clinical approach to the classification of deafness may not be helpful to the understanding of the pathology. Where a multiplicity of causes exists, as in deafness, we can appreciate the value for the clinician of the primary distinction between conductive and perceptive deafness. To see that this distinction is not always complete, we have only to bear in mind such lesions as acute otitis media extending to the labyrinth, and otosclerosis. The picture of acute inflammation following bacterial infection is a pathological entity, and its clinical effects depend on anatomical considerations. Otosclerosis is another pathological entity with varying clinical effects or none, depending, as far as is known, on the site of the lesions.

No deliberate use is therefore made in this work of the terms conductive or perceptive deafness. The classification is based on pathology, including that of the origins of profound childhood deafness, rather than the customary prenatal, perinatal and postnatal. Mainly these are due to microbial infection and genetic and inherited conditions, but not entirely so. It has therefore seemed rational to classify the causes as infections, further classified under the classes of microbial life; inherited diseases, inborn errors of metabolism and chromosomal anomalies; toxic causes, prematurity.

Neoplasia may affect hearing when metastasis (Friedmann and Osborn, 1965) invades the temporal bone, or by the development of acoustic nerve tumours.

The pathology of some forms of deafness remains obscure even where the aetiology seems clear, for example, in deafness following intra-uterine infections, such as syphilis and virus diseases, or the deafness associated with endemic goitre. Nor is it known whether deafness associated with exacerbations of rheumatoid arthritis is rheumatoid in its pathology or merely due to salicylates. The reasons for this obscurity are that human post-mortem material is hardly ever available, either because the disease, such as rheumatoid arthritis, is not usually fatal or because a condition such as late-onset deafness due to congenital syphilis remains hidden in the patient's personal history even if diagnosed at some time in his life, and is inherently unlikely to be in the case notes at the time of death. Nor perhaps does the general pathologist always realise the rarity of certain conditions within the temporal bone, and in this way important material may be lost.

Nevertheless, Fraser (1964) was impressed by the amount of descriptive histopathology of many inherited and other syndromes involving particularly the inner ear, and refers to many excellent reviews of the subject 'particularly in the German language'. He points out that the correlation between pathological clinical and genetical findings is surprisingly good, in recessively inherited deafness the changes being uniformly of the type first described by Scheibe (1892). There is degeneration of the organ of Corti, involving mainly the basal coil, with abnormalities of the tectorial membrane, stria vascularis and spiral ganglion. The saccule is also affected.

Considering the undoubted difficulties of differentiating between pathology and post-mortem change in the parts of the membranous cochlea, the similarities noted by Fraser might in part be due to the long interval between death and autopsy: in animal work either intravital fixation is insisted on for histological examination, or dissection and fixation within minutes of decapitation if the structure of the organ of Corti is to be seen at all resembling its structure during life. Temporal-bone sections nevertheless do give valuable information in other respects, provided that the autopsy follows refrigeration and is not delayed over twenty-four hours, as for other tissues

To be of further value, either glutaraldehyde or osmic acid 1·2 per cent solution should be injected through the foramen ovale as soon as is practicable after death. The only complete examination of the entire spiral organ is by the method of Engström (1966) following Retzius (1884), which uses phase-contrast microscopy of a surface view of the rows of hair-cells.

The prevalence of all forms of deafness is variously estimated: as late as 1960 Polish authors (Bystranowska *et al*.) attributed many cases of deafness in childhood to typhoid, dysentery and diphtheria, and in African countries meningococcal meningitis is still not uncommon. In the United Kingdom, Fraser estimated the population of deaf schools to be as in table II. These percentages are also

Table II

Genetic causes	Recessive	%
	With retinitis pigmentosa	7·5
	goitre	3·0
	abnormal ECG	1·0
	Others	26·0
	Dominant	
	With pigmentary anomalies	2·5
	Without pigmentary anomalies	10·0
	Sex-linked	1·5
Congenital malformations		2·5
Acquired	Prenatal	6·0
	Perinatal (including excess of prematurity)	10·0
	Post-natal	30·0
		100·0

equivalent to actual numbers per 100,000 live births in the general population.

Three main lines of investigation are possible for a pathologist. One is the collection of temporal bones from cases where there is some reason to suppose the findings will be abnormal, such as in Alport's syndrome, herpes zoster affecting the stato-acoustic nerve, and so on.

A second approach is the routine collection and examination of infant temporal bones: many infant deaths are associated with abnormalities such as congenital heart disease, and it might be expected that other abnormalities would be found in these cases. The state of the organs of hearing has not been described in many quite common developmental anomalies, for example the Arnold–

Chiari syndrome, which are of unknown aetiology, and of which some have been suspected of viral rather than genetic causation. Abortion material may also be of value.

The third line of approach is the attempted simulation of human disease in animals: all stages of otitis media due to any organism could be studied. Where the laboratory animal differs from man in response to certain pathogens, this line is of limited value. Nevertheless, much useful information has been derived from this approach.

A fourth line of approach is the serological survey of groups of patients suffering from (for example) sensorineural hearing loss to determine prevalence of a condition such as late-onset deafness due to congenital syphilis. To some extent this may be an approach to the assessment of the role of other congenital infections, namely toxoplasmosis and rubella in the causation of deafness.

At a time when obstetrics and paediatrics are saving lives which would have been lost only a generation ago, interest has been focused on the problems of the infant born of a difficult pregnancy, difficult labour or morbid inheritance. Two main clinical approaches are possible: the 'at risk' register, where the children who live are followed up, and the congenital malformation register, where all macroscopically abnormal infants are recorded and followed up. Neither method is suitable for a pathologist, whose investigations are mainly of those who do not survive, but whose information is an important supplement to both. Deafness for various reasons does not always receive the attention it should in either type of survey.

This work is based on a survey of the literature of the pathology of deafness, mainly compiled during the preparation of a London University Ph.D. thesis. The investigations into some aspects of the pathology of hearing loss, which formed the second part of that work, are published elsewhere, and are listed below.

'Investigation of ototoxicity of an antibiotic from *Micromonospora purpurea* (gentamycin)'. *Journal of Pathology* (1969), *98*, 129.

'The cytology of glue ear' (jointly with Rumy Kapadia), *Journal of Laryngology and Otology* (1969), *83*, 367.

'Late-onset hearing loss due to congenital syphilis: a serological survey in London, 1963–5', *International Audiology* (1968), 7, 302.

'The bacteriology of acute otitis media: an analysis of laboratory findings in infections of the ear, nose and throat in 1962–4', *Journal of Laryngology and Otology* (1970), *84*, 283.

'The effects of experimental infection of the guinea-pig with *Toxoplasma gondii* with special reference to transmission across the placenta'.

'Pathogenicity of *Toxoplasma gondii* and *Treponema pallidum* on introduction to the adult guinea-pig bulla'.

'Pathogenicity of *Toxoplasma gondii* and *Treponema pallidum* for the developing chick otocyst' (jointly with E. S. Bird).

'Liability of certain groups of congenital malformation and childhood illness to infections which may lead to deafness: the histopathology of middle and inner ear.'

References

Bystranowska, T., Kus, J., Osuch, T., and Wojnarowska, W. (1960), *Otolaryng. Polsk. 14*, 443.
Engström, H., Ades, H.W., and Andersson, A. (1966), *The Structural Pattern of the Organ of Corti*, Almqvist & Wiksell, Stockholm.
Fraser, G.R. (1964), *J. Med. Genet. 1*, 118.
Retzius, G.M., *Das Gehörorgan der Werbelthiere, Morphologisch-histologische Studien*, vol. I, 1881; vol. II, 1884; Stockholm.
Scheibe, A. (1892), *Arch. Otol.* (N.Y.), *21*, 12.

II The development of the embryo and the chromosomal anomalies

'By the 1930's Vogt had known that mobilisation and deployment of the cellular envelopes, tubes and sheets was the fundamental stratagem of early vertebrate development. . . . The theory of Spemann, that differentiation in development is the outcome of an orderly sequence, of specific inductive stimuli, led to the idea of search for the chemical properties of the inductive agent to find out why the amino-acid sequence of one enzyme or organ-specific protein should differ from the amino-acid sequence of another. The relative capabilities of the responding tissue were emphasised repeatedly, but only at theoretical level, for "competence" did not lend itself to experimental analysis.

'It is not now believed that a stimulus external to the system on which it acts can specify the primary structure of a protein, that is, convey instructions that amino-acids shall assemble in a given order. Embryonic development at molecular level must be an unfolding of pre-existing capabilities, an acting-out of genetically coded instructions' (P. B. Medawar).

The chromosomes carry the coded instructions, and may give rise to several kinds of genetic anomaly by failure of normal processes of division in cell multiplication. This may result in more than the normal complement of forty-six chromosomes in twenty-two pairs plus the X and Y pair (Tijo and Levan, 1956), or other genetic anomalies. The twenty-three pairs differ in appearance, and can be identified using the standard nomenclature.

Two broad categories of chromosomal abnormality have now been worked out, the autosomal (trisomies) and the gonosomal disturbance, according to the groups of chromosomes involved. Both are discussed later in this chapter.

The human embryonic life is usually held to be the first eight weeks. It is during this period that most 'environmental' factors are at work, whether infections, toxins, drugs or other factors. By the

end of eight weeks from the date of conception, usually taken as
14 days from the date of the last menstrual period, the embryo has
all its organs. Some differentiation remains, but growth is the main
foetal activity.

If a timetable of embryonal development is known, much time
can be spared in obtaining and analysing information about maternal conditions which are alleged to play a part in the causation
of foetal abnormality. Some events, such as a maternal infection or
exposure to a new drug, can be eliminated on grounds of date
alone, as the affected organ will have been fully formed by then.
Only malformations produced by the degeneration of already fully
formed structures can occur after development is complete. The
defect of an hereditary disorder is present from conception, but
cannot make itself known until the date for normal completion of
an organ is passed.

*The morphological mechanisms in the development of malforma-
tions*

These may be classified as follows (Millen, 1963):

1. Cessation of development before it is completed, developmental
   arrest.
2. Failure of normal developmental processes, agenesis or aplasia.
3. Excessive development, hyperplasia.
4. Aberrant development.
5. Failure of normal degeneration.
6. Secondary degeneration of normally developed structures.

Probably developmental arrest is the most important, and such a
failure can be dated as not later than the normal time of completion:
for example, if the palate and the facial processes are normally
fused at nine weeks, later events can be ruled out as having aetiological importance in either of these defects.

The second month of gestation is extremely crowded with events
and milestones of development: many malformations may then be
expected to occur together. Millen quotes anencephaly, cyclopia,
cleft palate and visceral anomalies as frequently associated. The
critical period for the limbs appears to be from the fourth to the
sixth weeks for the arms, and the fourth to eighth weeks for the

legs. Millen states that Lenz believed that the critical period for the administration of thalidomide is between the twenty-seventh and thirty-third days after conception.

Millen gives a useful timetable of human development, from which the extracts in table III are taken.

Table III

Age (days)	Size (mm)	
18	–	Neural plate and groove
26	3	Closure of anterior neuropore
		Arm buds appear
28	3·5	Closure of posterior neuropore
		Leg buds appear
24	3·0	Optic vesicles
27	3·3	Posterior neuropore. Ventral horn cells
31	4·3	Anterior and posterior nerve roots appear
24	3·0	Auditory placode
28	3·5	Otocyst cut off
42	13	Pinna forming
49	20	Cochlear duct, semi-circular canals
63	35	Fusion of palate completed

The development of foetal cochlear canals

Ormerod (1960) summarises the development of the human cochlea in greater detail as follows.

Fourth or fifth week: separation of otocyst from the structures of the neural crest. It forms two lobes; one will form the cochlea. The cochlea at first consists of the cochlear duct only, which by *six weeks* is a short tube lined with epithelium within primitive mesenchyme. It is a curved tube: it grows and completes the first turn at *seven weeks*. The scala vestibuli and scala tympani still consist of primitive mesenchyme, all within a cartilaginous capsule. At *nine to ten weeks* the full two and a half turns are developed, and the height of the cochlea is 3 mm; by the *fifth month* the height is 6–7 mm.

Differentiation of the cochlear duct epithelial lining begins about *eight weeks* in the base. By *twelve weeks* the future organ of Corti is apparent, and the tectorial membrane.

By *four months* hair-cells of inner spiral sulcus have formed in the basal turn, but are represented by a ridge of sensory cells at the apex.

By *six months* development is complete and the cochlea is ready to function.

The development of the middle ear

The whole development of the middle ear and auditory ossicles is dealt with fully by Bast and Anson in their classic *The Temporal Bone and the Ear*.

The resolution of the tympanic mass of mesenchyme has been described as a most intriguing problem by Guggenheim *et al.* (1956), who considered that a study of mesenchyme resorption in infancy was long overdue. Kelemen (1958) considered that the nature of new-born otitis (Schwarz, 1931) could not be settled without further understanding of this subject.

Judgment of foetal age

Head circumference and brain weight have been regarded as having a higher correlation with gestational age than any other common anthropometric measurement such as length or weight (Parmelee *et al.*, 1964). This is because these are largely unaffected by malnutrition. They are no use, however, in infants affected by congenital rubella or chromosomal abnormalities. In over-weight children of diabetic mothers the brain is near normal in weight for gestational age (Naeye and Kelly, 1966). For a full and useful account of brain development and reaction to malnutrition at vulnerable periods of growth, see Davison and Dobbing's *Applied Neurochemistry*.

Chromosomal anomalies

Mosaicism is an anomaly which can arise at any time during embryonic development, by the inclusion of both members of a chromosome pair in a daughter cell, or when one member lags at any phase and becomes effectively lost. In such ways, individuals may come to possess certain stem lines and clones with a different genetic constitution. This is obviously important when the sex-chromatin is involved. In a human with an XO/XX combination the phenotype is female, but is associated with gonadal dysgenesis. An XO/XY mosaic may be associated with either phenotype.

Other gonosomal disturbances are results from non-disjunction during oogenesis or spermatogenesis.

Klinefelter's syndrome, XXY, of which the characteristics are:

> phenotypically male
> gynaecomastia
> excess 17-Keto steroids
> aspermatogenesis
> sex-chromatin positive, i.e. Barr bodies

Turner's syndrome, XO:

> phenotypically female
> sexual infantilism
> pterygium colli and low-set pinnae
> cubitis valgus
> sex-chromatin negative, i.e. no Barr bodies
> liability to middle-ear disease

Superfemale, XXX:

> phenotypically female
> sex-chromatin positive
> usually mentally retarded

Trisomies

A great many syndromes have now been attributed to trisomies, and other chromosomal aberrations. As more facts accrue it becomes clear that, for the majority, more than one chromosomal alteration may be involved in the same syndrome. For example, Down's syndrome, which was initially identified as trisomy 21 by Lejeune *et al.* (1959), has now been reported associated with seven single-cell lines all involving trisomy 21, with some modification, and further, seven more reports where mosaicism also is present, again involving trisomy 21 (Baikie, 1965). With regard to the search for a 'genetic marker' for chromosome 21, Shaw and Gershowitz (1962) found some evidence that it may carry the ABO blood group locus, and Brandt (1963) that it may carry the locus for galactose-1-phosphate-uridyl transferase in the blood. Jerome (1962) suggests there may be an abnormality of tryptophan metabolism, and mongoloid individuals are known to secrete increased β-amino-isobutyric acid.

As chromosome 22 cannot be identified with certainty from 21, cases of trisomy 21–22 without the features of mongolism are often ascribed to 22. Some at least have muscular hypotonia.

The trisomies include:

1. Group 21–22–Y trisomy or translocation, resulting in Mongolism (Langdon-Down's syndrome).
2. Group 16–18.
3. Group 13–15.

1. *Mongolism* The suggestion that this syndrome (Down's syndrome) might be due to an abnormal chromosomal number was first made by Waardenburg in 1932 (Gairdner, 1965) and by Bleyer two years later, as a result in both cases of knowledge of consequences of abnormal number in other species: cytogenetics did not have techniques of human chromosome analysis available at that time so the suggestion progressed no further then. Special weight in diagnosis of mongolism should be given to palmar dermal ridges (Walker, 1957; Uchida and Soltan, 1963). Next most reliable, where diagnosis is in doubt, are increased acetabular-pelvic angles (Caffey and Rose, 1959). Naturally, microcephaly, short stature and mental retardation should be present.

2. *17–18 trisomy* (Edwards *et al.*, 1960; Patau, 1960). Trisomy E (Hecht *et al.*, 1963). Malfunction of nervous system. The characteristics are:

> low-set, malformed ears
> receding jaw, micrognathia
> cardiac anomalies
> abnormal palmar creases
> flexion contracture; 'surrender position' of hands, overlapping by index finger of others
> short big toes
> longest survival reported: twenty-three months (Weiss *et al.*, 1962)

No genetic marker is yet established, but Bühler *et al.* have found a defect of thyroxine synthesis in a child who is partially monosomic for the 17–18 group.

3. *Trisomy 16*   One case (Lewis *et al.*, 1963) described in a woman of 59, who also had precocious senility, osteoporosis and calcification of soft tissues (Lewis, Hymann, MacTaggart and Poulling, 1963).

4. *Trisomy 13–15*   (Patau *et al.*, 1960). Trisomy D[1]

  cerebral defect
  anophthalmia: absence of olfactory bulb and tracts
  cleft palate and harelip, and low-set ears
  polydactyly and trigger thumbs
  capillary haemangioma
  cardiac defect
  apparent deafness (see Patau *et al.*, 1961)

Becak *et al.* (1963) report two cases of 13–15 trisomy with general-ised analgesia but without the list above in which the only other anomaly present was slight mental retardation. Huehns *et al.* (1964) found one to six anomalous nuclear projections in neutrophil poly-morphs. One child had survived five years. 'No certain case of mosaicism has been reported', but Atkins and Rosenthal (1961) have described a case which Smith *et al* (1963) consider a possibility. The genetic marker may be persistent Gower-2 and gamma-4 haemoglobins.

  Deafness has been identified with a known chromosomal anomaly in group 13–15 trisomy (trisomy D, Patau *et al.*, 1960), in Turner's syndrome (Szpunar and Rybak, 1968), and in trisomy 18 (Kos *et al.*, 1966). Trisomies 13–15 and 18 are mentioned further on p. 32. Trisomy 17–18 (Edwards *et al.*, 1960) (trisomy E) has low-set malformed external ears: one probable example of this was examined and found to have normal middle and inner ear structure in spite of other congenital abnormalities.

  The hearing of mongols (Langdon-Down's syndrome, trisomy 21) is generally held to be acute, but of four cases examined two had purulent acute otitis media, one with excess protein in the labyrinth, and two had excess fluid and polymorphs in the middle ear not amounting to frank clinical otitis media.

The inborn errors of metabolism (see Duncan, 1964, table 51).

None of the inborn errors of metabolism is so far known to result in deafness.

References

Atkins, L., and Rosenthal, M.K. (1961), *N. Eng. J. Med. 265*, 314.
Baikie, A.G., in *Recent Advances in Paediatrics*, ed. Gairdner, G. (1965), Churchill, London.
Bast, T.H., and Anson, B.J. (1949), *The Temporal Bone and the Ear*, Thomas, Springfield, Ill.
Becak, W., Becak, M.L., and Schmidt, B.J. (1963), *Lancet, 1*, 664.
Brandt, N.J., Froland, A., Mikkelsen, M., Nielsen, A., and Tolstrup, N. (1963), *Lancet, 2*, 700.
Bühler, E.M., Bühler, U.K., and Stalder, C.R. (1964), *Lancet, 1*, 170.
Caffey, J., and Ross, S. (1956), *Pediatrics, 17*, 642.
Davison, A.N., and Dobbing, J. (1968), *Applied Neurochemistry*, Blackwell, Oxford.
Duncan, G.D. (1964), *Diseases of Metabolism*, fifth edition, Saunders, London.
Edwards, J.H., Harnden, D.G., Cameron, A.H., Crosse, V.M., and Wolff, O.H. (1960), *Lancet, 1*, 787.
Guggenheim, P., Clements, L., and Schlesinger, A. (1956), *Laryngoscope, 66*, 1303.
Hecht, F., Bryant, J.S., Motulsky, A.G., and Giblett, E.R. (1963), *J. Pediatr. 63*, 605.
Huehns, E.R., Lutzner, M., and Hecht, F. (1964), *Lancet, 1*, 589.
Jerome, H. (1962), *Bull. Soc. Med. Hôp. Paris, 113*, 168.
Kelemen, G. (1958), *Arch. Otolaryng. 68*, 547.
Kos, A.O, Schuknecht, H.F., and Singer, J.D. (1966), *Arch. Otolaryng. 83*, 439.
Lejeune, J., Gauthier, M., and Turpin, R. (1959), *C. R. Acad. Sci. Paris, 248*, 602.
Lewis, F.J.W., Hymann, J.M., MacTaggart, M., and Poulling, R.H. (1963), *Nature*, Lond. *199*, 404.
Lundin, L.G., and Gustavson, K.H. (1962), *Acta Genet. 12*, 156.
Medawar, P.B. (1967), from 'A biological retrospect' in *The Art of the Soluble*, Methuen, London.
Millen, J.W. (1963), *Develop. Med. Child Neurol. 5*, 343.
Naeye, R.L., and Kelly, J.A. (1966), *Pediatr. Clin. N. America, 13*, 849.
Ormerod, F.C. (1960), *J. Laryng. 74*, 919.
Parmelee, A.J., Jr., Stern, E., Chervin, G., and Minkowski, A. (1964), *Biol. Neonat. 6*, 309.
Patau, K., Smith, D.W., Therman, E., Inhorn, S.L., and Wagner, H.P. (1960), *Lancet, 1*, 790.
Patau, K., Therman, E., Smith, D.W., and Inhorn, S.L. (1961), *Hereditas, 47*, 239.

Shaw, M.W., and Gershowitz, H. (1962), *Am. J. Hum. Genetics*, *14*, 317.
Schwarz, M. (1931), *Arch. Ohr. Nas. Kehl. 129*, 1.
Smith, D.W., Patau, K., Therman, E. Inhorn, S., and De Mars, R.I., *J. Pediatr. 62*, 326.
Szpunar, J., and Rybak, M. (1968), *Arch. Otolaryng. 87*, 52.
Tjio, J.H., and Levan, A. (1956), *Hereditas*, *42*, 1.
Uchida, I.A., and Soltan, H.C. (1963), *Pediatr. Clin. N. America*, *10*, 409.
Walker, N.F. (1957), *J. Pediatr. 50*, 19.
Weiss, L., Digeorge, A.M., and Baird, H.W. (1962), *Am. J. Dis. Child*, *104*, 533.

III The development, blood supply and metabolism of the inner ear

The membranous cochlea is situated within the bony otic capsule, itself developed from cartilage during foetal life. It achieves adult size before birth. The details of this development are described by Bast and Anson (1949). Deriving from precartilage, the periotic labyrinth of fibrous tissue and fluid spaces separates the coiling cochlear epithelial tube and vestibular system from the bony capsule.

The growth of the bony otic capsule and of the auditory ossicles is complex (and the stapes undergoes modifications during development which make it unique). These all develop in cartilage. (The only membrane bones of the region are the tympanic ring and the squamous part of the temporal bone, both of which continue active growth into adult life, and the bony cochlear modiolus.) All three types of cartilaginous bone are present: perichondrial, endochondrial and intrachondrial, the last being unique to the otic capsule and the footplate of the stapes.

Perichondrial bone formation follows maximal cartilage growth, the cells enlarging, the matrix calcifying and the perichondrium becoming an epithelial layer recognisable as periosteum, and more vascular. Vascular osteogenic buds grow into the cartilage mass and form the network of *endochondrial bone*. At first this is a weak bone, and contains marrow spaces. Osteoclasts erode the calcified cartilage matrix in the bony trabeculae, and osteoblasts rebuild a strong cancellous bone. The later development of perichondrial bone is to the formation of compact lamellar bone.

Fourteen ossification centres exist, arising in relation to nerve terminations, and only when the cartilage has achieved its maximum size. The vascular pattern follows the centres. The intrachondrial bone of the otic capsule develops in the ossification centres: unlike the endochondrial bone, where the osteogenic buds excavate calcified cartilage, and replace it with marrow and ultimately the cancellous bone, osteogenic buds here are highly cellular and lay down bone within the cartilage lacunae from which necrotic cartilage cells have disappeared. Thus intrachrondrial bone may contain islands of cartilage matrix: the bone itself is endochondrial in type, and marrow may be present.

In the child, vitamin D is essential for absorption of calcium and normal bone growth: its absence produces the deformed epiphysis of rickets, and in the adult osteomalacia may result. Vitamin A appears to play some part in the growing bone metabolism, in so far as Mellanby (1938) found that puppies on an otherwise adequate diet developed bony overgrowth at the base of the skull and the vertebral foramina if they received no vitamin A.

Bone metabolism

In the adult this is maintained by adequate calcium and phosphate intake. The thyroid hormone thyrocalcitonin inhibits removal of calcium from the skeleton, thus acting as a parathormone antagonist, and suppresses excessive osteoclastic activity. To some extent oestrogens do the same. Osteoporosis may result from failure of these mechanisms in the general skeleton. Osteoblastic activity is promoted by pituitary growth hormone, androgens and anabolic steroids. Fluoride also may lead to osteopetrosis, and it is thought that osteoporosis is less common in areas where fluorosis is endemic. One of the early effects of fluoride administration is an osteomalacic picture following high serum alkaline phosphatase levels, later followed by calcification of the newly formed osteoid tissue.

The arterial supply to the bony otic capsule is from the external carotid system. The ascending pharyngeal branch reaches the petrous temporal bone, dividing into meningeal and *inferior tympanic* branches. The latter supplies the areas of the ossification centres 1, 2 and 4 (Bast and Anson), the fissula ante fenestram and the tympanic anastomosis. The occipital artery sends two branches to the otic capsule; the *posterior meningeal* supplies the dura round the endolymphatic sac, ossification centre 10, and the endolymphatic duct; the *recurrent mastoid* artery supplies the capsule of the posterior semi-circular canal and the region of the mastoid process. The *stylomastoid* artery (a branch of the posterior auricular) supplies the stapedius muscle, ossification centre 3 and the tympanic plexus, which further supplies centres 5, 7 and 8, and possibly accessory centres 11, 12 and 13. The *accessory stylomastoid* (also from the posterior auricular) supplies the facial canal and the lateral semicircular canal. The *subarcuate* artery supplies the superior semi-circular canal (centre 10) and the intervening region to the lateral canal. This artery alone among those supplying the bony labyrinth arises from the basilar arterial system.

Two small branches of the internal carotid artery supply the mucosa of the middle ear and the eustachian tube, while the middle meningeal artery sends branches to the facial nerve, the tympa-num, the tensor tympani muscle and the small bones of the middle ear.

Unlike the bony labyrinth, the membranous labyrinth receives its blood supply from an end-artery, the internal auditory artery, which is a branch of the anterior inferior cerebellar and thus from the basilar artery. Within the internal auditory meatus this artery divides into three, one to the saccule, utricle and semicircular canals, the second to the eighth nerve cochlear ganglion cells and the bony periotic capsule of the scala tympani, and the third to the bony capsule of the scala vestibuli and to the stria vascularis. There is no anastomosis between the two arterial supplies.

The illustrations in Nabeya's paper (1923) show that the venous drainage is not entirely parallel to the arterial supply.

The presence of vascular shunts in otosclerosis (Rüedi, 1965) and the effects of vascular pathology are mentioned in chapters later.

Stria vascularis

The development of the cochlear duct is fully dealt with by Bast and Anson. By the twelfth week of foetal life, Reissner's membrane is a simple columnar epithelium, flattening after the fourteenth week. In the basal turn first, the outer wall of the coiled cochlear duct is lined by a layer of slightly differentiated cells by the fifteenth week. Later it resembles a glandular epithelium, sometimes known as the glands of Shambaugh. This layer rests on the vascular tissues, the stria vascularis. This network is more easily understood with the diagram of Smith (1951) in mind (also reproduced in Best and Taylor's *Physiological Basis of Medical Practice*, eighth edition).

Nachlas and Lurie (1951) have reviewed the structure and func-tions of the stria vascularis. The authors concluded from animal

work that although structural changes in the organ of Corti were
accompanied by changes in the stria, the reverse was not necessarily
true, as in acoustic trauma. Thus no obvious constant relationship
could be established, and the authors' three possible types of function of the stria remain:

> Secretion
> Excretion
> Mechanical

Whilst most writers concede a secretory function, it seems not im-
probable that both secretion and absorption might occur—a state of
affairs not unknown in mammalian physiology, viz. the renal
tubule.

The structure of the normal guinea-pig stria vascularis, not well
illustrated in the paper of Nachlas and Lurie, is described as a
surface row of epithelial cells, separated during development of the
embryo from underlying tissue by a basement membrane, and
blood vessels developing beneath this (Shambaugh, 1907). The
adult form is not really described in this paper but the illustration
suggests a deeply staining layer of fairly tall cuboidal cells superficially, with connective tissue beneath, containing capillaries. There
is a line at which cleavage from the spiral lamina is easy to comprehend.

The relationship between the function of the stria and the circulation of endolymph is not wholly understood. Stacy Guild (1927)
traced precipitated prussian-blue granules from the cochlear duct to
the base of the cochlea and then on to the saccus endolymphaticus. A
few granules, however, were found in the stria. Adlington (1967)
has recently discussed the function of the saccus endolymphaticus
as a 'drain'.

Membranes of the inner ear and their significance

The ionic constituents of the fluids found in the channels in the
cochlea are of course important in relation to conduction of impulses. Other factors need consideration, such as the metabolism
of the hair-cells, their source of oxygen and other substances, and
the enzyme systems involved which release energy.

1. Ionic constituents of cochlear channel fluids, and their origins
Smith, Lowry and Wu (1954) showed that endolymph in the guinea-
pig contains a potassium concentration of 140–160 mEq/l, and 12–
16 mEq/l of sodium, whereas the perilymph contains 130–150
mEq/l sodium and 4–5 mEq/l potassium, thus resembling extracellular fluids and cerebrospinal fluid. The endolymph resembles
intracellular concentrations, and has been associated with the
requirements of conduction of impulses. The classical theory of
membrane potentials of Hodgkin, Keynes *et al*, was based on
differences of this calibre within and without nerve fibres. Citron,
Exley and Hallpike (1956) proved similar differences in concentrations in the cochlea of the cat, and Rauch and Köstlin (1958) in
man.

Naftalin and Harrison (1958) formed the hypothesis that ions
must penetrate Reissner's membrane, which separates the scala
vestibuli from the scala media. Diffusion potentials would result
from this penetration, and would appear in the endocochlear potential. Reissner's membrane is two-layered; earlier electro-physiologists
held that it was impermeable both to ions and to water. Electron-
microscopy has shown its structure of inner epithelial cells containing microvilli, vesicles, mitochondria and organelles, suggesting
considerable metabolic activity (Bairati and Iurato, 1964).

The source of water and ions and protein within the cochlear channels must ultimately be the bloodstream. The richest vascularisation
of the cochlea is in the region of the stria vascularis and the spiral
ligament. Rauch (1966) illustrates this from a guinea-pig cochlea by
Maas' technique of vascular injection.

Rauch (1966) investigated the possibility of 'flow' by an elegant
technique of injection with 'labelled' (isotopes of) sodium and potassium into the scala vestibuli basalis, and rapid freezing-fixation
after a given time. This was designed to make possible removal of
uncontaminated specimens of perilymph and endolymph from
every turn. He found that ^{29}Na appeared in the endolymph at ten
seconds, and ^{42}K appeared three times as fast in spite of the high
concentration gradient against this. Injection of these substances
into the scala tympani did not affect the endolymph, unless some
accidental flow had occurred over the helicotreme, suggesting the
impermeability of the basilar membrane.

To exclude the possibility of vascular uptake of the radioactive substances from the vessels in the lateral wall of the scala vestibuli, and rapid secretion from the stria vascularis, these experiments were repeated in a newly decapitated guinea-pig. The same rapid transport was obtained, provided injection followed decapitation within one to two minutes. At three minutes, decrease in ion-transport was found, which suggests that oxygen is required.

Rauch found that membrane-blocking substances, particularly kanamycin, blocked this transport.

The stria vascularis is likely to have as high an oxygen consumption as the cells of the retina: the cells are rich in mitochondria, particularly the dark apical cells. It is known to have sluggish blood flow. Rauch considers that little free oxygen would be left for diffusion in consequence of these factors. Rauch suggests that oxygen reaches the hair-cells and cortilymph via the spinal fluid flow along the spinal nerves. He found that Na^{24} injected into the facial canal reached the scala tympani via the cochlear duct within two minutes, but its concentration was ten to fifteen times higher in the cortilymph.

2. Possible sources of energy in the cochlear fluid channels   Carbohydrate metabolism produces energy in living animals: glycogen and glucose are particularly important sources. Glucose, transportable and readily utilised, is not a storable form, and its metabolism is particularly important in the brain where there are no carbohydrate stores.

Oxidisation of glucose yields thirty-eight molecules of ATP for one molecule of glucose. Anaerobic breakdown by glycolysis to lactic acid yields merely two molecules of ATP (Adenosine triphosphate).

ATP is essential for many metabolic processes, including the maintenance of normal relationships between intra- and extracellular electrolytes. The mitochondrion is the site of its formation: 95 per cent of the energy utilised by cellular activities is derived from the inter-action of oxygen with the electron-transport system of the mitochondrion. Breakdown products of fat protein and carbohydrate metabolism interact on the folded inner membrane with oxygen. The attribution of high energy output to a cell, such as a muscle-cell contracting, or a nerve-cell conducting impulses must always be supported at cellular level by evidence of mitochondrial function.

There are in fact three ways or metabolic schemes to store energy in the form of 'high-energy phosphate bonds'. Nerve metabolism does not differ from other tissues in this respect, all three are present and may be used.

1. Glycolysis. The Emden–Meyerhoff pathway.
2. Krebs' tricarboxylic cycle.
3. Electron-transport system.

1. Glycolysis is anaerobic, and only releases a small amount of ATP; glycolysis breaks down into pyruvate or to lactic acid.

2. The Krebs cycle breaks down the lactic acid to CO_2 and water, and requires oxygen to do so.

3. The oxygen unites with the hydrogen from the pyruvate, by means of the electron-transport system, which contains coenzymes (cytochromes and flavoproteins).

There is no doubt that all these possibilities exist in nerve tissue. Oxygen consumption and respiratory quotient indicate that the major substrate in the release of energy is probably not glucose: it remains unknown according to Boyarski (1966).

Human perilymph

Disc electrophoretic studies of the human perilymph (Palva and Raunio, 1967) have shown that pre-albumin, albumin, transferrin and haptoglobin bands are present in human serum, cerebrospinal fluid and perilymph. Large-molecule substances, such as group-specific proteins, gamma-globulins, and β_1-lipoproteins were weakest in the perilymph.

Two weak bands in the pre-albumin region were found in perilymph but not in serum or CSF. There was no evidence of fibrinogen.

Enzyme analysis showed by demonstrating lactic dehydrogenase activity that perilymph was an actively secreted fluid.

The eighth nerve

The eighth nerve cochlear division can be seen on leaving the
brain-stem as a myelinated nerve until it reaches the osseous spiral
lamina of the cochlea.

Within grey matter the axis cylinders are enclosed only by a
plasma membrane: the myelin sheath is acquired on leaving the
grey matter. It is a lipid material, and varies in thickness. It does
not cover autonomic nerve fibres, only those of somatic and cranial
nerves, which are usually larger fibres than the autonomic, and of
faster conduction. It may be the function of the myelin to insulate
the impulse conducted along the fibre. At a node, where the myelin
is thin, the neurilemma is highly permeable to ions, and it is
thought that the conduction of an impulse is 'saltatory', leaping
from node to node. The neurilemma covers the myelin and con-
stitutes the sheath of Schwann. Each internodal segment of the
sheath consists of one Schwann cell. At the node of Ranvier the
neurilemma dips downwards to the axon, for at this point, about
every millimetre, the myelin is absent.

Nerve fibres are myelinated first in the sensory pathways, and it
is believed that the time of myelination of a given tract coincides
with its first function. The spinal posterior columns (fourth and
fifth months of human foetal life) are followed by the spinocere-
bellar tracts, and the motor pathways come later; the pyramidal
tracts are not complete until the age that the child walks. Fibres of
association myelinate last.

Degeneration of a peripheral nerve may in certain circumstances
be followed by regeneration. This depends on the integrity of the
myelin sheath. Within the central nervous system there is no regeneration. Nor do we expect regeneration of fine, highly specialised
nerve endings, nor of end organs.

Techniques for visualising the fine nerve endings and their course
to the different rows of hair-cells have been described by Engström
et al. (1966), using freshly prepared zinc iodide. Nomura and
Kirikae (1967) used silver staining and an acetyl cholinesterase
method. Nomura and Schuknecht (1955) and Ishii, Murakami
and Balogh (1967) have also contributed to these methods.

References

Adlington, P. (1967), *J. Laryng. 81*, 759.
Bairati, A. and Iurato, S. (1964), in Rauch, S., *Biochemie des Hörorgans*, Stuttgart, p. 17.
Bast, T.H., and Anson, B.J. (1949), *The Temporal Bone and the Ear*, Thomas, Springfield, Ill.
Boyarski, L. (1966), in chapter 2 of Best, C.H., and Taylor, N.B., *The Physiological Basis of Medical Practice*, eighth edition, Livingstone, Edinburgh and London.
Citron, L., Exley, D., and Hallpike, C.S. (1956), *Brit. Med. Bull. 12*, 101.
Engström, H., Ades, H.W., Andersson, A. (1966), *The Structural Pattern of the Organ of Corti*, Almqvist & Wiksell, Stockholm.
Guild, S. (1927), *Amer. J. Anat. 39*, 1.
Hawkins, J.E. (1966), in chapters 17–19 of Best, C.H., and Taylor, N.B., *The Physiological Basis of Medical Practice*, eighth edition, Livingstone, Edinburgh and London.
Ishii, T., Murakami, Y., and Balogh, K. (1967), *Ann. Otol. 76*, 69.
Mellanby, E. (1938), *J. Physiol. 94*, 380.
Nabeya, D. (1923), *Acta Scholae Med. Kioto, 6*, 1.
Nachlas, N.E., and Lurie, M.H. (1951), *Laryngoscope, 61*, 989.
Naftalin, L., and Harrison, M.S. (1958), *J. Laryng. 72*, 118.
Nomura, Y., and Kirikae, I. (1967), *Ann. Otol. 76*, 57.
Nomura, Y. and Schuknecht, H.F. (1965), *Ann. Otol. 74*, 289.
Palva, T. and Raunio, V. (1967), *Ann. Otol. 76*, 23.
Rauch, S. (1966), *J. Laryng. 80*, 1144.
Rauch, S., and Köstlin, A. (1958), *Pract. Oto-rhino-laryng.* (Basel), 20, 287.
Rüedi, L. (1965), *Laryngoscope, 75*, 1582.
Shambaugh, G.E. (1907), *Z. f. Heilk. 53*, 312.
Smith, C.A. (1951), *Laryngoscope, 61*, 1073.
— (1957), *Ann. Otol. 66*, 520.
Smith, C.A., Lowry, O.H., and Wu, M.L. (1954), *Laryngoscope, 64*, 141.

IV Congenital malformations

In a paper entitled 'Definition and classification of human malformations' read at a study group on clinical research in human malformations at Liverpool in 1963, Davison says these are usually regarded as 'those morphological anomalies which are already present at birth and can be recognised macroscopically'. This would exclude anomalies recognisable only by biochemical or histological methods, the abiotrophic traits, the effects of metabolic anomalies only manifest later in life, and deafness. Sometimes anomalies are excluded because of determination by single gene substitutions or chromosomal abnormalities. 'This is helpful,' writes Davison, 'at least in aetiological studies in that each of these will have its specific familial pattern and incidence and the removal reduces a part, however small, of the heterogeneity in origins.' In studying a range of anomalies, if those with specific causes can be picked out it may be possible to look more clearly at the pattern of the remainder. This was the view taken by the Registrar-General's sub-committee on nomenclature and classification of congenital malformations, though the opposite view was taken by the comparable U.S. committee.

Methods of collecting information on prevalence

A system of coding requires transmissibility to simple punch cards: at least six malformations should be recordable for one child. The problem of adjacent combinations or rarities which could not be directly coded is dealt with by the use of 'further specified' or 'not further specified'.

One such system is that used in the Liverpool Congenital Malformations Registry. The punch card (fig. 2) and the classification list (table IV) have been in use for the Liverpool area since 1960. The method of collection of data is simple. Midwives on the district

GUY'S HOSPITAL, S.E.1

Name.............................., aged............of.........................

........................., has been delivered in this hospital and has been advised to attend her

local infant welfare clinic.

Date of delivery:

Particulars of labour:

Perineum

Loss

Duration of labour

Puerperium:

Condition on discharge:

Other information:

To the Medical Officer of Health,

Borough of.....................................

Date of discharge:

Weight: at birth: lbs.   ozs. ;

on discharge: lbs.   ozs.

Condition on delivery:

Feeding:

Other information:

Signed...

Date.. 19......

Fig. 1(*a*). The 'at risk' register.

If any abnormality occurred during pregnancy, labour, or puerperium, the child may be at risk of deafness or developmental abnormality.

Did any occur? Please state YES or NO.   If 'Yes', please ring appropriate number below:

Genetic: Family history of deafness, blindness, etc.   1

Pre-natal: Rubella or other virus infection in first sixteen weeks of pregnancy   2
Blood incompatibilities, e.g. Rhesus sensitisation   3
Hyperemesis   4
Ante-partum haemorrhage   5
Severe illness necessitating chemotherapy or major surgery in early months of pregnancy   6
X-ray other than chest x-ray   7
Thyrotoxicosis   8
Diabetes   9
Toxaemia of pregnancy   10
Other complications of pregnancy, e.g. pyelitis   11
Any psychiatric illness   12

Peri-natal: Prolonged or difficult labour   13
Birth weight under 4 lbs. Gestation less than thirty-six weeks   14
Birth asphyxia   15
Prolonged poor sucking   16

Post-natal: Jaundice   17
Convulsions   18
Respiratory distress, cyanotic attacks   19
Any congenital abnormalities   20

Fig. 1(b). Reverse of Fig. 1(a).

fill in and post a simple form, stating date, address, malformation(s). This information is coded and punched on receipt. Later, further inquiry may be necessary. Registrars in maternity and general hospitals notify the Registry similarly. Periodically the clerk who files the information visits other hospitals and receives names of children who are attending with, for example, congenital heart disease, and who should be added to the register: the Liverpool Dental Hospital yields, for example, previously unregistered cases of cleft palate of all types. In Liverpool, congenital malformations are notifiable diseases: this gives a further check via the Public Health Department on the completeness of the returns.

Table IV Liverpool list of abnormalities

1. Anencephaly and iniencephaly.
2. Spina bifida, meningocele.
3. Hydrocephalus.
4. Hypospadias.
5. Syn/polydactyly.
6. Congenital heart disease.
7. Mongols.
8. Exomphalos.
9. Cleft palate.
10. Cleft lip.
11. Intestinal obstruction.
12. Kidneys and ureters.
13. Skeletal.
14. Jaw, tongue, gums and pharynx.
15. Congenital dislocated hip.
16. Central nervous system (other).
17. Eyes.
18. Ears and branchials.
19. Skin and subcutaneous tissue.
20. Lungs, trachea, larynx, diaphragm.
21. Talipes.
22. Genital tract (excluding hypospadias, UDT, hydroceles).
23. Skull.
24. Metabolic.
25.
26. Umbilicus (excluding exomphalos).
27. Endocrine.
28. Pancreas, liver, biliary tract.
29. Muscles.
30. Congenital tumours.
31. Bladder and bladder neck.
32. Conjoined twins and monsters.
33. Chromosome abnormalities.
34. Multiple (34) and syndromes.
35. Miscellaneous.

The Liverpool system differs from the 'at risk' register. The Guy's Hospital 'at risk' register is kept by the midwifery superintendent, who informs the Medical Officer of Health of the borough in which the mother resides by ringing relevant information on the standard form (fig. 1).

Although either system could probably be used by an otologist who was interested in the appearance of deafness not due to simple otitis media in such children, neither has necessarily a wide enough net to include such conditions as might be of particular importance in the aetiology of deafness. For example, a mother who has had rubella during the first trimester of pregnancy would be included in an 'at risk' register; only if her baby had an obvious defect such as cataract would it be included in the Liverpool scheme unless or until it was diagnosed as having congenital heart disease. We know from the Public Health Laboratory Service rubella working party's prospective survey into the effect of rubella in pregnancy that some pregnant women have a fourfold rise in antibody titre to rubella: in a prospective survey such as this, the infants can be followed up in any way required. It would indeed now be possible to examine selected children from this survey with regard to hearing, though the two years' clinical examination would mostly have elicited deafness of the grosser sort.

McDonald (1958) attempted to relate maternal health during pregnancy with subsequent defect in the child. She carried out a prospective survey of 5,295 women in the Watford–St Albans area in 1952–55. There were sixty-eight (2 per cent) spontaneous abortions, sixty-three still-births (2 per cent) and thirty-five (1 per cent) neonatal deaths. Only forty-seven of the still-births and twenty-seven of the neonatal deaths were not associated with major congenital defect.

In all, 122 infants had congenital defects (3·8 per cent of all progeny) fifty major (1·5 per cent) and seventy-two minor (2·3 per cent). Deafness is not one of the defects recorded, possibly because age of final follow-up of infant preceded possible diagnosis. No difference in maternal health during pregnancy was found between those who delivered premature infants, infants with minor defects, and those whose infants were normal. The mothers of infants with major defects had a higher incidence of febrile illness early in pregnancy, as had those who aborted.

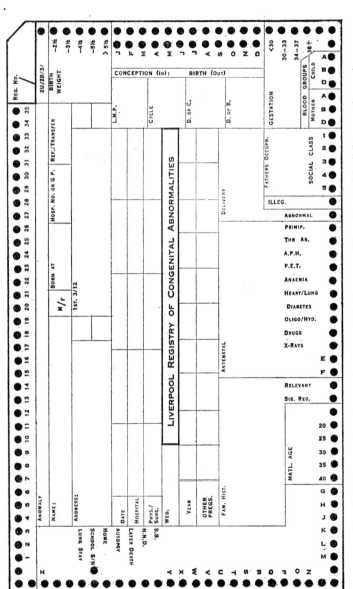

Fig. 2. Liverpool registry of congenital abnormalities (see table IV): punch card.

Fraser (1964) has estimated deafness associated with congenital malformations, often multiple, at 2·5 cases per 100,000 live births, and 2·5 per cent of cases of profound childhood deafness. He includes examples of the Treacher-Collins syndromes, some dyscephalies, and middle-ear and bony labyrinthine deformities. The fact that rubella has widespread effects on the developing foetus suggests the possibility of other maternal infective processes playing a similar role in the development of congenital anomalies not considered to be inherited.

Investigations of families of affected children are not likely to be productive of relevant information. A prospective survey of maternal virus infections during pregnancy is now in hand by the Public Health Laboratory Service, and if it includes assessment of hearing in its final clinical follow-up of the resulting infants, some useful information may be acquired.

The Mondini and Scheibe types of defect

Probably the following malformations are more properly considered as inherited disorders. The histopathology is described by Nager (1925). *Mondini* published the description of a cochlear malformation in 1791. 'The aqueductus was wide and the vestibule a little bigger than normal. The semi-circular canals were normal. Of the cochlea, only the first one and a half coils were normal. Above them was only a cavity with a slender rest of the modiolus in the middle.' This is quoted by Guffarth (1936) and Jensen (1967). (See also Gussen, 1968.)

Mygind (1893) found ten temporal bones with this malformation in hereditary deafness in the Ibsen–Mackeprang collection. Guffarth (1936) found six cases, which had histological descriptions, in the world literature. Fraser (1964) regards the hereditary status as 'unclear'.

The *Scheibe* lesions, with normal bony labyrinth, are usually found in recessive inherited deafness. They include degenerated organ of Corti, atrophic stria vascularis, abnormalities of the tectorial membrane and spiral ganglion, and saccular changes. Fraser considers the *Michel* type of malformation possibly similar to that described radiologically by Everberg *et al.* (1963) in the Klippel–Feil syndrome, but see also chapter v on the damage caused by thalidomide, which includes aplasia.

Congenital atresia of the ear has been reviewed by Altmann (1949, 1955).

Chromosomal anomalies of hearing

Trisomy syndromes 13–15 (D) and 17–18 (E) Kos, Schuknecht and Singer (1966) have described the histological appearances of three temporal bones from two cases of trisomy 13–15 and one of trisomy 18. They refer to Mottet and Jensen's (1965) previous description, where there were no abnormal findings.

Kos *et al.*'s case 1 has cochlear and saccular abnormalities on both sides. In the basal turn of the cochlea the organ of Corti is missing or replaced by fibrous tissue. The stria vascularis is atrophic or absent and Reissner's membrane missing. In the remainder of the cochlea, Reissner's membrane is depressed and collapsed onto the organ of Corti and the stria vascularis. The spiral ganglion is normal. The saccular wall is collapsed and lies upon the macula.

Case 2 (one side) is very similar, but in addition part of the bony cochlea is missing.

Case 3 (trisomy 18): the right ear presents abnormalities in the inner ear, the ossicles and the tensor tympani. The cochlea, how-ever, presents an incompletely developed spiral modiolus. Some spiral ganglion cells lie in the internal auditory meatus. The organ of Corti, the saccular and the utricular maculae appear normal. (The child responded to sound.)

The left ear shows a missing utriculo-endolymphatic valve. The cochlea is flattened, and bony partition between the middle and apical turns is missing. There is almost complete absence of the ganglion cells of the spiral ganglion. There are a few at the extreme base of Rosenthal's canal. There are a few fibres in small bundles which enter this modiolus and pass to the organ of Corti. These are probably efferents from the olivo-cochlear bundle. The hair-cell population of the organ of Corti is described as normal. The stria vascularis is normal.

Kos *et al.* note that these abnormalities are similar to those described by Scheibe (1895), but recently Schuknecht, Igarashi and Gacek (1965) have described cochlea-saccular degenerations as due to inherited anomaly, to viral disease, or to ageing, though these are not exclusive.

Schwartz *et al.* (1964) have discussed trisomy 17–18 in relation to malformation of the ear. Fraser (1964) points out that casual testing of a child's hearing, when mental retardation is also present, cannot definitively exclude deafness.

Other chromosomal anomalies are recorded, including gonosomal non-disjunctions such as the XXXXY cases, the eleventh case to be reported being described by Joseph, Anders and Taylor (1964). No mention of deafness is made, but the multiple defects present include short neck, smallness of size for age, widely set eyes, epicanthic folds, patent ductus arteriosus; all of which suggest it should be excluded. The only illness recorded of the mother during pregnancy was toxaemia: she also had a long labour, delivering by breech presentation after fifty hours. In some ways these cases resemble Down's syndrome, in which no hearing defect is reported. One feature of the trisomy 18 cochlea described by Kos *et al.* resembles the Mondini malformation, namely the scala communis. The temporal bone of one probable case of trisomy 17–18 seen by the author showed no abnormality.

Defects of the nervous system

Hydrocephalus and meningomyelocoele   There is no recognised association between hydrocephalus and deafness. McNab (1965) discusses sight in this condition and concludes it would be defective, terminally, when intraventricular pressure was so high as to produce degenerative changes in the region of the basal ganglia and the lateral geniculate body. Papilloedema is not present in hydrocephalus if the block in the ventricular system or the subarachnoid space prevents the transmission of increased pressure to the orbital portion of the subarachnoid space. This argument seems likely to apply to the sheath of the eighth nerve. In one severe case seen by the author, dilated lymphatics accompanied the seventh nerve within the temporal bone. The bone beneath the dura showed pressure necrosis. Within the bony otic capsule, there was no abnormality such as endolymphatic hydrops. Increased protein was present in all channels, but autolysis was present (this case was still-born, and probably died *in utero* some days previously).

Hydrocephalus, though not associated with meningocoele, develops in 50 per cent of cases of myelomeningocoele by three months of age, 35 per cent showing some degree of hydrocephalus at birth. Commonly, the cause of the hydrocephalus in these cases is the Arnold–Chiari malformation, where an elongated fourth ventricle opens into the spinal subarachnoid space below the foramen magnum. The Arnold malformation is the herniation of a part of the cerebellum into the spinal canal: the Chiari, the elongation of the fourth ventricle, see also Willis (1962).

Three cases of meningomyelocoele with Arnold–Chiari malformation, complicated by meningomyelitis, were found by the author to have complete cochlear destruction due to inflammation. Unfortunately, no material was obtainable from anencephaly, or from a Klippel–Feil syndrome.

Anencephaly is probably due to a primary arrest of the closure of the neural tube. Morgagni (1761) noticed abnormally small adrenal glands associated with it, and it is now believed that this is secondary to the anterior brain defect, as these glands develop normally till the fifth foetal month. Females outnumber males. The eyes and external ears are usually well-developed (Willis, op cit., p. 148.)

Iniencephaly is a gross malformation incompatible with post-natal life, again commoner in female foetuses. It amounts to a Humpty-Dumpty figure. It is probably due to failure of development in the third week or earlier. The eyes are developed.

Gilmour (1941) considered the Klippel–Feil malformation, associated with deafness, a mild form of the same anomaly. Potter (1953) has depicted an intermediate condition. Other authors have described examples with associated alimentary malformations. (Willis, op. cit., 157–159.) See also Ballantyne (1904), Gilmour (1941) and Potter (1953).

Werdnig–Hoffman disease Progressive infantile muscular atrophy, a disease of the lower motor neurones, is distinct from amyotonia congenita (see Walton, 1957) and from the muscular dystrophies. Willis classifies this as an abiotrophic disorder of the central nervous system and includes it in a chapter on inborn metabolic and allied disorders. The pathology of the abiotrophies is a degeneration of groups or tracts of neurones, with accompanying gliosis. The term abiotrophy was used by Gowers, and the accepted meaning

is of a degeneration within the central nervous system, first manifesting itself in post-natal life. These are not, therefore, properly
included with congenital malformations. See Walton (1957), Willis
(1962). Of two cases seen by the author, in one the temporal bone
showed otitis media, and the other had lymphocytic infiltration of
the stria vascularis, suggesting a virus infection. There was also
lymphocytic infiltration of the middle-ear mucosa.

Skeletal defects

Treacher-Collins' syndrome   This is one of the mandibulo-facial
dysostoses, and includes deformities of the facial bones, outward
and downward slope of the palpebral fissure, bilateral notching of
the outer third of the lower eyelid with deficiency of lashes on the
medial third. Deformities of the ear, both external and middle,
may be present; none was present in the only specimen available
for examination by the author. This syndrome may include
micrognathia.

The defect appears to date from the seventh week of foetal
life. The deafness is predominantly conductive, and this inheritance
is dominant. There is marked variability and deafness is not always
present. See Harrison (1957). It should be remembered that
micrognathia may be a feature of Still's disease.

Cleft palate   Deafness may be associated with cleft palate. The fact
that the human palate is formed by maxillary coalescence as late as
the tenth embryonic week allows for unusually prolonged opportunity for arrest by harmful influences (Willis, 1962). It is thus a
frequent malformation, and it is therefore surprising, as Holborow
(1962) points out, that the deafness—which he found in half his
patients—has found so little mention in the literature. There was,
however, absolute agreement that the type of deafness was conductive. Skolnik (1958) states that 2 per cent of all cleft palate patients
have a congenital anomaly of the ear: the series included 401
patients, 39 per cent of whom were deaf, and 45 per cent of whom
had 'definite pathology', by which he meant clinical ear disease.
Many of the other anomalies were not confined to the head and neck
but included limb deformities.

Among the causes of deafness, Holborow discusses infection,

lymphoid hyperplasia, tubal stenosis, palatal dysfunction. As a result
of experimental work with dogs, he concluded that malfunction of
the tensor palati was largely responsible, owing to weakness of the
muscle; before closure of the cleft, because of the presence of the
defect; after closure, because of damage at operation. He advised
against tonsillectomy and adenoidectomy.

The heart

Many malformations are known, and the heart is not infrequently
affected in multiple malformations (Willis, pp. 181-2) as in rubella,
which is a congenital cause of deafness. Study by the author of the
temporal bones from fifteen children with congenital heart disease
showed but four cases of acute otitis media, one of which had progressed to a destructive panotitis. Five of the cases had a slight to
moderate inflammatory exudate in the middle ear. One had excess
lymphoid tissue in the mastoid and petrous marrow. This is a high
rate of infection and may be due to prolonged illness. No malformations of the Scheibe or Mondini type were found.

Tracheal stenosis or atresia

The larynx or trachea may be occluded by a cartilaginous mass,
epithelialised on upper and lower surfaces. Lung development may
be normal.

Tracheo-oesophageal fistula is frequently accompanied by oesophageal atresia, but rarely, if ever, by tracheal atresia. (Willis,
op. cit., p. 194.)

Material from these conditions showed no structural cochlear
abnormality, but cases were liable to infections of the middle ear.

References

Altmann, F. (1949), *Arch. Otolaryng. 50*, 759.
— (1955), *Ann. Otol. 64*, 824.
Ballantyne, J.W. (1904), 'The embryo', *Manual of Antenatal Pathology.*
Davison, C. (1963), *Develop. Med. Child Neurol. 5*, 340.
Everberg, G., Ratjen, E., and Sorensen, H. (1963), *Brit. Jl. Radiol. 36*, 562.
Fraser, G.R. (1964), *J. Med. Genet. 1*, 118.

Fraser, J.S. (1922), *J. Laryng. 37*, 13, 57, 126.

Gilmour, J.R. (1941), *J. Path. Bac. 53*, 117.

Guffarth, F.X. (1936), *Das pathologisch-anatomische Bild der hereditär-degenerativen Innerohrschwerhörigkeit bzw*, Taubheit, Tübingen.

Gussen, R. (1968), *J. Laryng. 82*, 41.

Harrison, M.S. (1957), *J. Laryng. 71*, 597.

Holborow, C.A. (1962), *J. Laryng. 76*, 762.

Jensen, J. (1967), *J. Laryng. 81*, 27.

Joseph, M.C., Anders, J.M., and Taylor, A.I. (1964), *J. Med. Genet. 1*, 95.

Kos, A.O., Schuknecht, H.F., and Singer, J.D. (1966), *Arch. Otolaryng. 83*, 439.

MacDonald, J.G., and Peckham, C.S. (1967), *Brit. Med. Jl. 3*, 633.

McDonald, A.D. (1958), *New Eng. J. Med. 258*, 767.

McNab, G.H. (1965), in *Recent Advances in Paediatrics*, ed. D. Gairdner, third edition, Churchill, London.

Michel, E.M. (1863), *Gaz. Med. Strasb.*, ser. 2, *3*, 55.

Millen, J.W. (1963), *Develop. Med. Child Neurol. 5*, 346 (see also *Develop. Med. Child Neurol. Symposium*, 1964, 6).

Mottet, N.V., and Jensen, H. (1965), *Amer. J. Cl. Path. 43*, 334.

Mygind, H. (1893), *Z. Ohrenheilk, 24*, 103.

Nager, F.R. (1925), *Z. Hals. Nas. Ohr. 11*, 149.

Potter, E.L. (1953), *Pathology of the Foetus and the Newborn*, Chicago.

Public Health Laboratory Service rubella working party (1967), *Brit. Med. Jl. 3*, 638.

Registrar-General's Sub-committee on Nomenclature and Classification of Congenital Malformations.

Scheibe, A. (1895), *Arch. Otolaryng, 24*, 280.

Schuknecht, H., Igarashi, M., and Gacek, R.R. (1965), *Acta. Otolaryng, 59*, 154.

Schwartz, M., and Becker, P.E. (1964), in Becker, P.E. (ed.), *Human Genetik*, Thieme, Stuttgart, pp. 248–345.

Siebenmann, F. (1904), *Grundzüge der Anatomie und Pathogenese der Taubstummheit*, Wiesbaden (see Fraser, J.S.).

Skolnik, E.M. (1958), *Laryngoscope, 68*, 1908.

Walton, J.N. (1957), *Proc. Roy. Soc. Med. 50*, 301.

Willis, R.A. (1962), *The Borderland of Embryology and Pathology*, second edition, Butterworth, London.

V Maternal disease during pregnancy and 'excess of prematurity'

Some infections, acute or chronic, bacterial, viral or protozoal, can cross the placenta. These are described in the chapters on infections.

This chapter is concerned with the effect on the hearing organs of the developing foetus of diabetes mellitus, toxaemia of pregnancy and hypertension. Hypothyroidism is dealt with in chapter VI. Drugs which can adversely affect the developing foetus include thalidomide, which is included in this chapter rather than with ototoxic drugs (chapter VII).

Deafness following rhesus incompatibility is also mentioned here, though its cause may be post-natal, and is certainly through the medium of high bilirubin levels damaging the cochlear nuclei. Cavanagh (1954), in following up eighty-two children who developed deafness, sixty-four of whom were anaemic enough to require transfusion in days when exchange transfusion was not commonplace, found twenty-eight with neurological impairment. Of those not transfused, one had severe deafness. Fisch and Osborn (1954) found that twenty-seven out of 891 children with congenital perceptive deafness had had haemolytic disease: twenty of the twenty-seven had other severe neurological disease.

Maternal diabetes and the ears of new-borns

Kelemen (1955–1960) described two foetal inner ears, and Jorgensen (1961) those of a full-term infant born of a diabetic mother, and Buch and Jorgensen (1966) described six more such infant temporal bones.

None showed signs of the PAS-positive deposits found in adult diabetic vascular striae, nor any pathological change such as haemorrhage, which could not be attributed to the pressures and anoxia of birth.

The placenta of Jorgensen's (1961) case, (*aet.* 27, who had been a diabetic since the age of 5) was described, at full term and after an uneventful pregnancy, as weighing 1200 g, large, oedematous, loose and lobular without infarctions. The infant became cyanosed soon after birth, and died at twenty hours. Post-mortem examination found nothing remarkable, except that the baby was a typical infant born of a diabetic mother: it weighed 3,750 g, length 53 cm, and had plump extremities, short neck and puffy skin.

The temporal bone histology showed:

Middle ear. Normally ossified ossicles. Some foetal mesenchyme, in which there had been small bleeds.

Inner ear. The bony labyrinth was everywhere fully developed and of normal appearance. Throughout the mesenchyme of the perilymphatic spaces there were engorged vessels and in several places small haemorrhages.

The organ of Corti and stria vascularis had marked degenerative changes, the neuroepithelial cells of the stria showing such disintegration that there was no demarcation from the connective tissue of the spiral ligament.

There was considerable tortuosity and engorgement of the walls of the scalae tympani and vestibuli, and no trace of Reissner's membrane. Modiolar vessels also were congested and tortuous.

In Kulchitzky-stained preparations the myelin sheaths were intact throughout. Jorgensen (1961) comments that the vascular and neuroepithelial changes could hardly have occurred during the twenty hours of life had they resulted from anoxia and pressures during delivery; further, they resemble the appearances in Kelemen's hysterectomy cases. He concludes that these represent pre-delivery pathology, destructive though they are, and are to be expected in the babies of diabetic mothers. However, haemorrhages are found commonly in all post-mortem examinations of still-born or neonatal death temporal bones (Buch and Jorgensen, 1966; Buch, 1966).

As these authors comment, there was no control series of post-mortems on infants without some trauma or asphyxia during labour, or even hysterectomy. Nor are there clinical tests to elucidate function of the vestibular and cochlear endorgans and nerves in a new-born child. But Buch and Jorgensen (1966) conclude that the changes are not really relative to the maternal diabetes mellitus, but more to stresses of late pregnancy and labour, although many of the foetuses were large and were delivered by caesarian section.

The largeness of 'diabetic' infants is not to be equated with maturity necessarily: these infants have large fat stores and may be premature by other criteria.

Full-term and premature new-born ears

The inner ear of new-born infants, including one case of endolymphatic hydrops in the cochlea of a newborn, has recently been investigated.

Buch and Jorgensen (1964) found haemorrhage most common in the internal auditory meatus. Perineural extravasates were found in fifty-eight of seventy-three new-borns, and intraneural in thirty-seven. The vestibular ganglion was often surrounded by extravasates, and the nerve cells here and in the spiral ganglion might be surrounded by red blood cells. Twelve infants had extravasated blood within the modiolus.

Within the membranous labyrinth, extravasation of blood was most common in the perilymphatic spaces, the cochlea being clearly more affected than the vestibular part. The scala tympani was involved twenty-five times, the scala vestibuli nineteen, and the cochlear duct five. The scala tympani had the more massive haemorrhages. Red blood cells were seen between the organ of Corti and the tectorial membrane.

In ten cases there was a degenerated organ of Corti and some were accompanied by an atrophic stria vascularis. The illustrations of Buch and Jorgensen's paper show that the preservation is not at fault: these are not due to post-mortem autolysis, even though, as they state, in Denmark it is not permitted to perform a post-mortem until several hours after death.

Analysed with regard to prematurity, thirty-nine labyrinthine haemorrhages were found in fifty-nine premature infants, and two in the fourteen of over 2,500 g birth weight.

Other evidence supports asphyxia and prolonged labour as causes of haemorrhage into the membranous labyrinth. Aurup (1959) has also shown that twins, especially the first-born and the smaller one, have a hearing impairment more often than would be expected statistically.

There was an excess of 'post-matures' among the infants in the Buch and Jorgensen (1966) series; predominantly in this group the stria vascularis was congested or atrophic.

One case in this series is clearly of endolymphatic hydrops, and the authors were unable to suggest an aetiology: the mother was severely anaemic and presented an inevitable abortion at about five to six months. The infant lived fifty-five hours. No aetiology was suggested.

Maternal hypertension and toxaemia

The hypertensive and the toxaemic mother tend to produce premature infants. No specific damage to the hearing organ has been recorded, but McDonald (1964) examined 1,028 children for deafness at 6–8 years whose birth weight had been 4 lb or less. Nineteen could not be traced, twenty-eight had died; of the original number, nineteen had severe or moderate perceptive deafness (1·8 per cent). Of those whose gestation period was less than thirty-three weeks, sixteen were deaf out of 387 children (twins *not* included), or 4·1 per cent, as compared with 0·6 per cent in 339 children of more than thirty-three weeks' gestation.

Clearly, birth weight is of significance only in relation to gestational age, as an aetiological factor in the background of perceptive deafness (McDonald, 1964). Many had had oxygen and antibiotics.

There was no suggestion that oxygen therapy of itself was harmful. Some suggestion that streptomycin was damaging was found. As Fraser (1961) points out, in premature infants renal function is immature and cannot prevent development of high drug and antibiotic levels in plasma, and ototoxic levels are possible in endolymph and cortilymph.

Thalidomide in pregnancy: effect on the development of the middle and inner ear

No damage is done by this drug to the human foetus if administered before the thirty-fourth or after the fiftieth day of pregnancy. Phocomelia is not seen after the forty-second day (Lenz, 1963). These are presumably days from the LMP, i.e. equivalent to nineteen to thirty-five post-conception days and twenty-seven days respectively.

Jorgensen, Kristensen and Buch (1964) have described a case of thalidomide-induced aplasia of the inner ear in a girl aged one month referred with deformity of the external ears, congenital heart disease and facial palsy. (Congenital total aplasia of the inner ear has been previously reported only by Michel (1863).)

The mother of this case had taken one or two tablets of 100 mgm of thalidomide at about twenty-five days after conception. This is the age at which Bast and Anson (1949) found the otocyst forming as an ingrowth from the ectoderm into the mesoderm, dorsal to the second branchial groove.

The findings were: no seventh or eighth cranial nerves, one rudimentary middle ear, with no cavity for the inner ear, and one slit-shaped middle ear, with normal drum malleus and incus, and head and limbs of stapes. There was no oval window or footplate, but there was a smooth-walled spherical cavity within an otic capsule. Microscopically, sensory and supporting cells were thought to be present, but no nerve cells or fibres.

Rosenthal (1963) and Barr and D'Avignon (1963) have reported also developmental anomalies of the external ear often associated with facial palsy. Everberg (1960) has described techniques for radiological identification of bony dysplasias in the temporal bone.

References

Aurup, R. (1959), *Nord. Med. 62*, 1303.

Barr, B., and d'Avignon, M. (1963), *Medicinsk. Rikstämma* (Stockholm).

Bast, T.H., and Anson, B.J. (1949), *The Temporal Bone and the Ear*, Thomas, Springfield, Ill.

Buch, Nils, and Jorgensen, M.B. (1964), *Arch. Otolaryng. 80*, 60 (newborn).

Buch, Nils (1966), *J. Laryng. 80*, 765–1006 (hydrops).

Buch, Nils, and Jorgensen, M.B. (1966), *J. Laryng. 80*, 1105.

Cavanagh, F. (1954), *J. Laryng. 68*, 444.

Everberg, G. (1960), *Acta Otolaryng. 52*, 47.

Fisch, L., and Osborn, D.A. (1954), *Arch. Dis. Child. 29*, 309.

Fraser, G.R. (1961), *Brit. Med. Jl. 2*, 1361.

— (1964), *J. Med. Genet. 1*, 1964.

Jorgensen, M.B. (1961), *Acta Otolaryng. 53*, 49.

Jorgensen, M.B., Kristensen, H.K., and Buch, N. (1964), *J. Laryng. 78*, 1095.

Kelemen, O. (1955), *Arch. Otolaryng. 62*, 357.

Lenz, W. (1963), International Conference on Malformations, reported by C.O. Carter in *Devel. Med. Child Neurol. 5*, 654.

McDonald, A.D. (1964), *Arch. Dis. Child, 39*, 272.

Michel, M. (1863), *Gaz. Med. Strasb.* ser. 2, *3*, 55.

Rosenthal, T. (1963), *Lancet, 1*, 724.

Symposium on Embryopathic Activity of Drugs held at University College, London, 1965, publ. 1967.

VI Hormones and deafness

Thyroid dysfunction

Thyrotoxicosis has no effect on hearing, but thyroid deficiency causes hearing loss. Two series of primary hypothyroidism in adults (Lerman, Murray, quoted by Means, De Groot and Stanbury, 1963) found that 30 per cent and 40 per cent were deaf, as were 26 per cent of Murray's fifteen further patients with pituitary hypothyroidism. Vertigo may also be an early symptom. The fact that deafness may be unilateral suggests that the cause is within the labyrinth. Poulsen (1966) has demonstrated doubling of numbers of mast cells in the labyrinthine connective tissues, and great increase in metachromatic substances in endolymph and perilymph in simulated myxoedema in guinea-pigs. The middle-ear mucosa and the connective tissue of the eustachian tube showed similar changes, but there was no sub-sarcolemmal accumulation of mucopolysaccharide in the muscles of the middle ear as in orbital muscles. Cases diagnosed as Ménière's disease (see also chapter xiv) should be investigated for hypothyroidism: Poulsen finds that those with a low basal metabolic rate improve both vestibular and cochlear function on thyroxine, and considers that the fluid and mesenchymal changes of hypothyroidism would be compatible with the endolymphatic hydrops reported (Hallpike and Cairns, 1938) in Ménière's disease. Audiologically, the deafness of adult hypothyroidism is generally considered as having a conductive element, but being mainly central in type (de Vos, 1963). Stephens (1970) has shown that the lesion is probably sensorineural, and proximal to the hair cells. All are agreed that it improves on thyroxine. The histopathology is reviewed by de Vos (1963). It is clear that the deafness of congenital hypothyroidism is more severe, and histologically intracochlear changes include thickened basilar membrane and reduction of eighth nerve ganglion cells (Albrecht, 1934; Lüscher, 1938). The pathology in four temporal bones from cases of goitre with deafness referred to by Fraser (1964) is confusing

(Manasse, 1909; Brock, 1920; Nager, 1925; Ormerod, 1960; de Vos, 1963). These cases illustrate the difficulty of interpretation of post-mortem material which may have undergone autolysis before fixation. Cases of Pendred's syndrome, which is *sporadic goitre* and perceptive deafness inherited together, may be apparently euthyroid. Fraser (1964) considered that a temporal bone from this condition had almost certainly not been examined histologically. The inheritance is recessive.

The possibility has been suggested that Pendred's type of deafness is due to a defect which also affects thyroxine synthesis to some extent. The deafness is related to a goitrogenic factor and the patient may not be hypothyroid. The goitre may well be small. Pendred's cases fail to convert inorganic to organic iodine, probably owing to the absence or low level of one particular enzyme. Means, De Groot and Stanbury classify familial hypothyroidism on the basis of possible enzyme defects. Briefly, the synthesis of thyroxine is in several stages. The iodide is taken up and trapped, and must be oxidised before it can be incorporated in the tyrosyl residues in thyroglobulin. Means, De Groot and Stanbury consider that one enzyme is responsible for each of the groups of inherited hypothyroidism, which they classify as follows:

1. Defect of iodine uptake.
2. Failure to convert iodide to organic form, with Pendred's syndrome as a less severe sub-group.
3. Failure to couple mono- and diiodotyrosine into triiodotyrosine and thyroxine.
4. General lack of iodotyrosine deiodinase.
5. Abnormal iodinated peptide in plasma, instead of thyroxine.

The goitre of Pendred's syndrome is sometimes wrongly considered malignant because of the marked pituitary stimulus to the thyroid gland.

Any form of hypothyroidism may be associated with a sensorineural deafness, which may not be severe, and may not appear till long after the onset of hypothyroidism or of Hashimoto's disease or after thyroidectomy.

The deafness of adult non-cretinous endemic goitre is sometimes associated with euthyroidism. Trotter (1960) considers that prenatal iodine lack may be responsible. Deaf-mutism is common in all alpine districts where iodine intake is low (Srinivasar, 1964).

Platybasia has been found in all x-rayed skulls of cretins in an endemic goitre region of Yugoslavia (Podvinec, 1966). Podvinec considers that platybasia represents a normal stage of foetal development which should not persist into post-natal life. It is known that the greater quantity of circulating thyroxine is required in athyreotic monkeys by the skeletal and nervous systems. It is considered that the foetus's own thyroid will be hypofunctional if maternal iodine intake is insufficient, and little transfer of maternal thyroxine occurs. This would account for euthyroid individuals with platybasia and hearing loss in endemic goitre districts, resulting from maternal inadequate iodine. (See also leading article in the *British Medical Journal*, 1958.)

In conclusion, the causation of deafness in hypothyroidism appears likely to be due to mucopolysaccharide accumulation in endolymph, perilymph and connective tissues of the labyrinth. As in other tissues the severity depends on the thyroxine level. The need for thyroxine is known to be high in nerve and other highly specialised tissues.

Other mechanisms may play a part in Pendred's syndrome and those endemic goitre cases who are euthyroid.

Nodular goitre and thyroid carcinoma and deafness have been reported by Elman (1958).

The parathyroid

One clinical case of primary hypoparathyroidism in which severe deafness developed during chilhood has been reported by Kendall (1965). The connection is not established.

Diabetes mellitus

The effect of diabetes on the adult ear (The infant ear, born to a diabetic mother, see chapter v; apparently familial diabetes mellitus and nerve deafness, see chapter viii.) Diabetes mellitus is a metabolic defect characterised by inadequate insulin secretion, and hence

by intermittently high levels of blood glucose. The main complications of the untreated or poorly stabilised diabetic state are:

1. Liability to autointoxication by ketones, resulting from inadequate metabolism of carbohydrate and fats: this will produce
   coma, accompanied by dehydration and death.
2. An abnormal liability to infections.
3. Neuropathy.
4. Retinopathy.
5. Vascular degenerative states more advanced than in age peers.

There are two types of diabetes: the severe type coming on in early
life, and that of middle-age, always associated with obesity.

The complications of diabetes affecting hearing are:

1. Inflammation Acute otitis media and mastoiditis in middle age
may be the first indication of the diabetic state of the patient. It has
no other singularities, but responds to treatment when the diabetes
is controlled. It will not be further discussed here.

2. Neuropathy Jorgensen and Buch (1963) investigated a series of
sixty-nine diabetics, chosen from young patients of long-standing
history, and concluded that twenty-eight of them had a progressive
bilateral perceptive deafness; some had an acute onset, with tinnitus
and vertigo. Where recruitment tests were carried out the lesion was
found to be cochlear. The vestibular part of the labyrinth did not
appear to be involved. One patient had a Bell's palsy. Fifty-eight of
this series were further subjected to tests of capacity for smell and
taste, and thirty-five had impairment, while twenty-four were
severely anosmic, but no changes were found for taste. Those
patients whose hearing was affected tended to have retinopathy,
but not those with disturbance of smell. It was assumed that the
pathogenesis of the hearing loss, which was commoner in the older
than the younger diabetics, was due to angiopathy.

Buch and Jorgensen (1966) quote the only histological descriptions
from Panse (1906), Witmaack (1907) and Voss (1931) but point out
that these have been criticised by Kindler (1955) on the grounds that
such severe changes as were found would be unlikely to be due to
prolonged diabetes in those so young. The changes in Witmaack's
case included reduction of the cells of the spiral ganglion.

Jorgensen (1961) described the pathology of temporal bones from a group of thirty-two diabetics dying in Copenhagen and Aarhus, their ages not stated. Changes were found in the vessels of the stria vascularis identical with angiopathy described by other authors in cases of late diabetic complications in kidneys, joints and nerves. These were, in addition to common changes of ageing, severe PAS-positive thickening of the capillary walls of the stria vascularis. Similar changes were sometimes found in the intraneural vessels of the facial nerve. Further, there was a progressive reduction of the ganglion cells in the basal part of the spiral canal and PAS-positive thickening of the basement membrane of the vessels of the stria vascularis: these are similar to the changes of old age (Jorgensen, 1961).

Jorgensen suggests that the Ménière-like syndrome from which some diabetic patients suffer may be due to haemorrhage from fragile capillaries in the stria vascularis.

Some of the new anti-diabetic drugs may be ototoxic or cause at least temporary deafness; see De Sa and Bhargava (1968) on R.94 (N. Benzine sulphonyl-n-isopropyl urea). No animal work or human pathology report has yet appeared.

Acromegaly

Richards (1968) has drawn attention to a statistically significant incidence of otosclerosis in a series of acromegalics. Deafness has previously been attributed to eustachian obstruction in these patients.

References

Albrecht, W. (1934), *Z. Hals Nas. Ohr. 36*, 262.
— (1944), *Z. Hals Nas. Ohr. 50*, 63.
Brock (1920), *Arch. Ohrenheilk. 105*, 135.
Buch, N.H., and Jorgensen, M.B. (1966), *J. Laryng. 80*, 1105 (ears, maternal diabetes).
Jorgensen, M.B., and Buch, N.H. (1963), *Acta Otolaryng. 53*, 351 (adult diabetic and hearing), 539 (smell and taste in diabetics).
De Sa, J.V., and Bhargava, K.B. (1967), *Acta Otolaryng. 64*, 537.
De Vos, M. (1963), *J. Laryng. 77*, 390.
Elman, D.S. (1958), *New Eng. J. Med. 259*, 219.

Fraser, G.R. (1965), *Ann. Hum. Genet. 28*, 201.

Fraser, G.R., Morgans, M.E., and Trotter, W.R. (1960), *Q.J.Med. 29*, 279.

Hallpike, C.S., and Cairns, H. (1938), *J. Laryng. 53*, 625.

Johnson, S. (1958), *Acta Otolaryng.* Supp. 140.

Jorgensen, M.B. (1961), *Arch. Otolaryng. 74*, 373 (diabetes).

— (1961), *Arch. Otolaryng. 74*, 164 (ageing).

Kendall, D. (1965), *Proc. Roy. Soc. Med. 58*, 1087.

Kindler, W. (1955), *Pract. Oto-rhino-laryng.* (Basel), *17*, 921.

Lerman, J. (1955), in *The Thyroid*, ed. S. C. Werner, Cassell, London.

Lüscher, E. (1938), *Schweiz. Med. Wiss. 68*, 835.

Manasse, P. (1909), *Z. Ohrenheilk. 58*, 105.

Means, J.H., De Groot, L.J., and Stanbury, J.B. (1963), *The Thyroid and its Diseases*, third edition, McGraw-Hill.

Murray, I.P.C. (1962), M.D. thesis, University of Glasgow.

Nager, F.R. (1925), *Z. Hals. Nas. Ohr. 11*, 149.

Ormerod, F.C. (1960), *J. Laryng. 74*, 919.

Panse, R. (1906), *Arch. Ohr. Nas. Kehl. 70*, 15.

Podvinec, S. (1966), *Medical Tribune*, 21 July.

— unpublished but reported at Turin conference.

Poulsen, H., in *Hormones and Corrective Tissue*, ed. G. Asboe-Hansen, Munksgaard, Copenhagen, 1966.

Richards, S. (1968), *J. Laryng. 82*, 1053.

Smith, J.F. (1960), *Q. J. Med. 29*, 297.

Srinivasar, S. (1964), *Lancet, 2*, 176.

Stanbury, J.B. (1963), *Recent Progress in Hormone Research, 19*, 547.

Stephens, S.D.G. (1970), *J. Laryng. 84*, 317.

Trotter, W.R. (1960), *Brit. Med. Bull. 16*, 92.

Voss, O. (1931), *Z. Hals. Nas. Ohr. 29*, 230.

Witmaack, K. (1907), *Z. Ohrenheilk. 53*, 1.

Leading article (1958), 'The skeleton and thyroid deficiency', *Brit. Med. Jl. 1*, 567.

VII Ototoxic agents

A list of drugs and substances which have been associated with deafness would include:

Aniline dyes	Mercury
Aconite	Morphine
Antipyrine	Nitrobenzole
Barbiturate	Novocaine
Benzene	Salicylate
Carbon disulphide	Scopolamine
Carbon monoxide	Strychnine
Caffeine	Streptomycin
Camphor	Viomycin
Chenopodium	Kanamycin
Chloroform	Gentamicin
Chloroquin	Polybrene
Ergot	Salvarsan
Hydrocyanic acid	Valerian
Iodine	Alcohol
Iodoform	Tobacco
Lead	

All but the antibiotics, frusemide, polybrene and ethacrynic acid are dealt with by Taylor (1937).

Polybrene

A polymeric quaternary salt, polybrene is known to be nephrotoxic (Haller *et al.*, 1962) and is reported by Ransome *et al.* (1966) as ototoxic.

Polybrene (Abbott) is hexadimethrine bromide; as a macromolecular substance it resembles Dextran, in that with increasing molecular size increases its toxicity. Its use is in counteracting the effect of heparin, which is used in haemodialysis to prevent coagulation in the extra-corporeal circulation. It has been preferred to protamine sulphate on the ground of less toxicity, but several dialysis units in London and Montreal have noted severe perceptive deafness and tinnitus following its use. This has so far not been reported in open-heart surgery. The pathological findings were: gross degeneration of the organ of Corti, degeneration of the stria vascularis, and some loss of cells from the spiral ganglion. Reissner's membrane appeared thickened, the endolymphatic sacs showed some disorganisation and ruptures. There was sub-epithelial oedema of the connective tissue of the cupulae and maculae. No PAS-positive deposits were found.

The ototoxic antibiotics

These are usually streptomyces products, and renal damage and hair-cell damage are reported for kanamycin (Engstrom *et al.*, 1966; Matz *et al.*, 1965), streptomycin and neomycin (Frost *et al.*, 1960; Friedman *et al.*, 1967). Kohonen (1965) adds framycetin, and Wright (1969) gentamicin.

Vionactan (Jelert, 1967, a clinical report only) is a streptomyces floridae isolate. It is tuberculostatic and just as ototoxic as, or more ototoxic than, other streptomyces which damage the hair-cells if high plasma concentrations are maintained.

Gentamicin   Wersäll (1967) has reported outer hair-cell damage, particularly in the basal turn of the cochlear in guinea-pigs on very high dosage such as 100–400 mgm per kg body weight daily in divided doses. He did not have the opportunity to estimate the renal function or histology of those animals that died with or without ototoxic signs.

Gentamicin is closely related to kanamycin and neomycin, and like these is a broad-spectrum antibiotic of considerable potential. It contains deoxystreptamine, as do kanamycin, neomycin and paramomycin. In addition, it contains two other amino-sugars, 2-amino-hexose and N-methyl-3-amino-D-xylose (Weinstein, 1967). Its close relationship to the streptomyces antibiotics suggest that vestibular and cochlear damage are not unlikely, as Cawthorne and Ranger (1957) has shown for streptomycin, and Leach (1962) for neomycin and other members of the group. Friedmann, Dadswell

and Bird (1966) have demonstrated by electron microscopy extensive vestibular and cochlear damage in the guinea-pig following the
administration of neomycin sulphate. Black *et al.* (1963) have
demonstrated damaged vestibular function in rat, cat and dog
following gentamicin administration. Lundquist and Wersäll (1967)
have demonstrated that the ototoxicity was greater than that of
streptomycin or kanamycin in guinea-pigs, in an electron micro-
scope study. Flandre and Damon (1967) have shown tubular renal
damage in rats. Although the doses used in these investigations
achieve higher blood levels than would normally be attained in
clinical use, it is considered that the presence of renal damage would
predispose to vestibular damage and deafness. Fraser (1961) has
commented on damage to the hair-cells of the foetus with a non-
functioning kidney by antibiotics administered to the mother.

Gingell and Waterworth (1968) have recorded blood levels in
normal human subjects and in uraemic and non-uraemic patients
receiving gentamicin. The manufacturers have advised that the
serum level should not exceed 10 μgm/ml. As Gingell and Waterworth point out, it is those patients with impaired renal function
who are most likely to benefit from the use of such an antibiotic
which can be effective in the treatment of chronic urinary infection. They have shown that in subjects with normal renal function
on 40 mg of gentamicin intra-muscularly, the highest peak level
in the serum was 4·1 μgm, clearly inadequate for *Ps. aeruginosa*. In
subjects with defective glomerular filtration, higher levels were
maintained for a longer period, which is satisfactory for the treatment of this chronic renal infection, but may allow toxic levels to
develop in other tissue fluids. This would include the fluid which
surrounds the organ of Corti.

An investigation planned with the critical range of dosage suggested by Lundquist and Wersäll's results in mind, demonstrated
the potential of gentamicin as an agent which may destroy the
hair-cells of the organ of Corti, which were directly examined using
Engström's surface preparation and phase-contrast microscopy
(Wright, 1969).

Quinine

Taylor (1937) considered that deafness might be produced in
the foetus if quinine were ingested by the mother, but Fowler

(1939) found no clinical evidence of this. Covell (1936) found hair-cell damage in guinea-pig foetuses—indeed, permanent changes can be ascribed to it. Taylor states that the number of neurons may be reduced. Two of Harrison's (1959) cases of congenital deafness in children followed their mothers' attempts at abortion with quinine.

Salicylates

Siberstein, Bernstein and Garfield Davies (1967) have shown that acute salicylate intoxication lowers the malic dehydrogenase activity in endolymph and perilymph. Hyperglycaemia occurs, and the endolymph and perilymph are both shown to have elevated glucose levels. Sodium, potassium and total protein concentrations are unaffected. No structural changes were found.

Salvarsan (atoxyl)

Reported by Miyamote (1931), who found collapse of Reissner's membrane in 50 per cent of guinea-pigs on toxic dosage, with atrophy of the stria vascularis. The ganglion cells and the organ of Corti also showed advanced changes. Taylor (1937) finds the question of eighth nerve damage unanswered.

Ethacrynic acid and frusemide

Mathog et al. (1970) have demonstrated hair-cell damage with these.

References

Black, J., Calesnick, D., Williams, D., and Weinstein, M.J. (1963), *Antimicrobial Agents and Chemotherapy*, p. 138.
Cawthorne, T., and Ranger, D. (1957), *Brit. Med. Jl. 1*, 1444.
Covell, W.P. (1936), *Arch. Otolaryng. 23*, 633.
Flandre, O., and Damon, M. (1967), Symposium on gentamicin, Geneva, 1966.
Friedmann, I., Dadswell, J.V., and Bird, E.S. (1966), *J. Path. Bac. 92*, 415.
Frost, J.O., Hawkins, J.E., and Daly, J.F. (1960), *Amer. Rev. Resp. Dis. 82*, 23.

Gingell, J.C., and Waterworth, P.M. (1968), *Brit. Med. Jl.* 2, 19.

Haller, J.A., Jr., Ransdell, H.T., Jr., Stowens, D., and Rubel, W.F. (1962), *J. Thorac. Cardiovasc. Surg. 44*, 486.

Harrison, K. (1959), *J. Laryng. 73*, 451.

Jelert, H. (1967), *J. Laryng. 81*, 317.

Kimura, E.T., Young, P.R., and Barlow, G.H. (1962), *Proc. Soc. Exp. Biol.* (N.Y.).

Kohonen, A. (1965), *Acta Otolaryng.*, Supp. 208.

Leach, W. (1962), *J. Laryng. 76*, 774.

Lundquist, P.G., and Wersäll, J. (1967), symposium on gentamicin, Geneva, 1966.

Mathog, R.H., Thomas, W.G., and Hudson, W.R. (1970), *Arch. Otolaryng. 92*, 7.

Matz, G.J., Wallace, T.H., and Ward, P.H. (1965), *Laryngoscope, 75*, 1690.

Miyamote, T. (1931), *Arbeit. Med. Universitat. Okayama, 2*, 412.

Ransome, J., Ballantyne, J.C., Shaldon, S., Bosher, S.K., and Hallpike, C.S. (1966), *J. Laryng. 80*, 651.

Siberstein, H., Bernsteon, J.M., and Garfield Davies, D. (1967), *Ann. Otol. 76*, 118.

Taylor, H.M. (1937), *Laryngoscope, 47*, 692.

Wersäll, J. (1967), symposium on gentamicin, Geneva, 1966.

Wright, I. (1969), *J. Path. 98*, 129.

VIII Deafness associated with familial disease

Arthur (1965) lists hereditary syndromes that include deafness. Many good references are also supplied on the occurrence of pigmentary disturbance and deafness in animals in this paper.

Danish *et al.* (1963) give the following list of multiple anomalies from a deaf population. Not all these are hereditary diseases. References are given here for those syndromes not referred to later.

1. Cogan's syndrome. (Keratitis and perceptive deafness not now thought familial) (see chapter x).
2. Lenticular abnormalities (probably Alport's syndrome).
3. Juvenile optic atrophy (Leber's). Gates (1946) considered the deafness independent in the one family in which it was associated.
4. Retinitis pigmentosa (Usher's syndrome).
5. Waardenburg's syndrome. Dominant.
6. Mental retardation (Pearson, 1912).
7. Endemic goitre (see chapter vi).
8. Non-endemic goitre (Pendred's) (see also chapter vi).
9. Nodular goitre and thyroid carcinoma (see chapter vi).
10. Friedreich's ataxia. Gates mentions one family which probably had independent deafness.
11. Myoclonic epilepsy. One (very) inbred family has familial deafness as well.
12. Huntington's chorea. Gates notes one family with independent deafness.
13. Subcortical encephalopathy. Deafness part of progressive lethal brain disease due to demyelination.
14. Osteogenesis imperfecta (Ekman–Lobstein) (Adair–Dighton) (Eddows).
15. Osteopetrosis. See Nelson's *Textbook of Paediatrics*, 1959 edition, p. 1240.
16. Osteitis deformans (Paget's disease of bone).

17. Laurence–Moon–Biedl retinitis pigmentosa, polydactyly, mental defect pituitary defect.
18. Neurofibromatosis (Gardner and Turner). One family where auditory nerve tumours presented in six generations.
19. Pulmonary stenosis (Lewis, S.M., Sonnenstick, B.P.G., Ibert, L., and Biber, D. (1958), *Am. Heart J. 55*, 458).
20. Jervell–Lange Nielsen. Cardiomyopathy (see this chapter).
21. Hereditary interstitial pyelonephritis (see Alport's syndrome, this chapter).
22. Hereditary nephropathy (see Alport's syndrome).
23. Wilson's disease (Everberg, G. (1957), *Acta. Scand. Psychiat. 32*, 307).
24. Periodic peritonitis (Mamou and Cattan (1952), *Semaine Hôp. Path. 28*, 1062.)
25. Ectodermal dysplasia. One family has hearing defect as well.
26. Retinal degeneration, obesity and diabetes mellitus (Alston, 1959).
27. Trisomic syndromes, Patau's group D1, 13–15, Edward's group E, 16–18. (These are not thought familial; see chapters II and IV).

Arthur adds:

28. Treacher-Collins (see chapter IV).
29. Hunter–Hürler (see chapter IX).
30. Cleft palate, though the deafness may often be conductive in type due to liability to infection and Eustachian obstruction (see chapter IV).
31. Klippel–Feil, though there is no obvious simple hereditary pattern.

To these should be added Cockayne's syndrome (Cockayne, 1936) and Wildervanck's syndrome of split hand and foot apparently of dominant inheritance associated with perceptive deafness. Fisch (1959) would add early greying of the hair and deafness, which he regards as separate from the Waardenburg trait. Febrile urticaria, inherited (probably dominant) amyloidosis and nerve deafness have been described by Muckle and Wells (1962), *q.v.* Otosclerosis (see chapter XI) is clearly a hereditary disease.

To these might be added many rare combinations of inherited

defects including deafness, such as the following culled by Fraser (1964) from the literature:

37. Retinitis pigmentosa, deafness; hypophosphataemia, glycosuria and rickets (Jackson and Linder, 1953).
38. Ataxia; progressive peripheral muscular wasting; perceptive deafness in childhood but no retinitis pigmentosa; metabolic block in steroid metabolism (Richards and Rundle, 1959).
39. Retinitis pigmentosa; deafness; gonadotrophic and ovarian hormones subnormal (Roberto and Carbonara, 1959).

There are of course families in which one or more abnormal inheritance may become manifest. All authors agree that there is an association between eye, ear, and the central nervous system during development. This need not imply more than disturbance at one stage of pregnancy leading to failure in subsequent development.

Those syndromes of connective tissue disease associated with deafness and which appear to be familial are mentioned in chapter x, e.g. myositis ossificans progressiva.

Dominant syndromes

Alport's syndrome (partially sex-linked dominant) This is a familial and uncommon disease of the kidneys associated with progressive perceptive deafness. Williamson's (1962) account of three further families presenting features similar to Alport's (1927) family does much to elucidate the syndrome. By 1962 it was known to affect twenty more families, with 250 affected individuals. It consists of:

Hereditary nephritis, probably by a partially sex-linked dominant trait, as males are more severely affected than females, though females transmit the gene to their offspring. The renal lesion presents early in life, as acute glomerulonephritis with haematuria, and albuminuria which is persistent. Affected males do not usually survive 30 years of age. The pathology of the kidney has been accepted as a chronic glomerulonephritis; there may be severe lymphocytic interstitial infiltration, so that Goldbloom *et al.* (1957) and Perkoff *et al.* (1958) have suggested that a recurrent pyelonephritis is the renal disorder. In some cases large numbers of lipid-containing foam cells were seen (Goldbloom *et al.*, 1957; Perkoff *et al.*, 1958;

Castleman, 1957). Robin *et al.* (1957) suggests that there may be two renal syndromes, the second a pyelonephritis inherited as a simple dominant. Williamson suggests that Løken *et al.*'s family may belong to this group.

Hearing disorder. This is always sensorineural, coming on at about 10 years of age, and progressive: it is less common in affected females than males. Williamson stated that no satisfactory histological evidence of the state of the inner ear was available, but since then Gregg and Becker (1963) described one case showing degeneration of the stria vascularis and the hair cells, especially in the basal coil, in a boy of 7½ years, with ocular lens rupture in one eye and later juvenile cataract formation in the other. The spiral ganglion, Reissner's membrane, basal membrane and other labyrinthine structures were normal. Another is described by Crawfurd and Toghill (1968). Hamburger *et al.* (1956) consider that the inheritance of the hearing disorder may be by partially recessive sex-linked gene, but Perkoff *et al.* (1958) consider it to be possibly linked with the renal lesion.

Perkoff *et al.*'s case 5, dying *aet.* 43, had foam cells in his kidney, and the temporal bone histology is described: 'There was hyperostosis at the tip of the cochlea and in other sites which could not be localised accurately, but other abnormalities were not noted. Unfortunately the stapes and oval window could not be identified because of the plane of the sections. In addition the cellular detail was poor, so the adequate evaluation of the organ of Corti was not possible. None of the foam cells which characterised the renal lesion in the patient could be demonstrated in the ear.'

The appearances in Crawfurd and Toghill's case included a cystic spiral ligament, and a dilated saccus endolymphaticus, containing two polypoid connective tissue projections and many hundreds of foam cells. Degeneration of the organ of Corti and collapse of Reissner's membrane, which could be autolytic changes, were also present.

Ophthalmic defects. Sohar (1956) describes congenital cataracts and spherophakia in his Israeli family. Arnott, Crawfurd and Toghill (1966) review the lens defects in the literature, and describe a new case, whose temporal bones are described in Crawfurd and Toghill (1968).

The incidence of Alport's syndrome is not known, but Williamson states that his three families accounted for 'more than a quarter of our cases of "acute nephritis" which still had abnormal urine at the six-month follow-up', which points to a higher incidence than would be suspected from published reports.

Krickstein *et al.* (1966) have shown that the renal foam cells contain cholesterol and phospholipid. They note that there is in some affected families a susceptibility to beta-haemolytic streptococcal otitis media. This is an interesting suggestion, in view of the connection between streptococcus pyogenes infections and acute glomerulonephritis. They describe renal pathology for thirteen unrelated families. They conclude that the most acceptable explanation of Alport's syndrome is a genetic defect, in an enzyme system affecting the known sites, possibly by leading to an accumulation of a toxic metabolic product, and stress that renal and auditory systems are similarly susceptible together to toxic antibiotics.

Waardenburg's syndrome The full syndrome described by Waardenburg in 1951 consists of wide separation of the inner canthi of the eyelids, and a broad nasal root, unequally coloured eyes, a white forelock and perceptive congenital deafness. The full manifestations are rarely seen; usually several or one or two of these are seen in a family carrying the trait. Another feature is congenital atresia of the oesophagus so that, as in Fisch's family (1959), some relatives were lost in early childhood of a wasting disease. McDonald and Harrison's cases included vitiligo of the forehead with the white forelock in a negro child, the inner parts of the eyebrows also being affected.

Fisch (1959) studied the deafness of the syndrome in some detail, and his paper includes a histopathological study by Friedmann. He considers it not so uncommon as was previously thought. He was able to collect eighty-one cases, and of these thirty-five were studied in detail.

Fisch considers the eyelid deformity to be the commonest, and that white forelock alone may not represent the Waardenburg trait, pointing out that the Dukes of Northumberland, the Percy family, have exhibited this trait for 500 years. The skull has a particular configuration so that 'Waardenburg'-afflicted children resemble one another, with large jaw, depressed nasal bridge and sometimes a metopic suture. Patchy pigmentation of the skin is sometimes noted, particularly in flashlight photography, which contains a large element of ultra-violet light.

One of the children with oesophageal atresia also had a large Meckel's diverticulum.

The temporal-bone histology in one of these cases showed absence of the organ of Corti in all turns of the cochlea, although the inner ear appeared to be fully developed, the maculae of the utricle and saccule were fully developed, and hair-cells were visible there. The vascular stria was normal. The spiral ganglion contained only a few ganglion cells, though bundles of nerve fibres were seen entering the basilar membrane in a fairly normal fashion. Examination of the brain showed no abnormality except that the cochlear root of the eighth nerve was thin and poorly myelinated.

Fisch considers that this pattern—i.e. absence of end-organ and peripheral neurone without disturbance of the central pathway—is not uncommon, particularly in malformations arising early in foetal life. In discussing the association of pigmentary defects with deafness he points out that the pigmenting cells of both choroid and iris are derivatives of the neural crest, which in itself is responsible for the developing otocyst. He further adds that skin pigmentation and the development of the functional hearing are protective, and usually, in all groups of mammals, develop about the same time.

Fisch suggests the phylogenetic 'median eye' is related to the area of pigmentary and skeletal abnormality.

This appears to be a dominant inheritance with varying expression and possibly low penetrance. A woman carrying the trait has a 50 per cent chance of giving birth to a child similarly affected. As one-third of those affected are deaf, such a child has a one in six risk of severe deafness.

Recessive

Cardio-auditory syndrome of Jervell and Lange Nielsen This is a recessive syndrome characterised by liability to fainting, or indeed sudden death, a very unusual electro-cardiogram with a prolonged QT wave, and profound perceptive deafness.

Jervell and Lange Nielsen (1957) described four affected sibs out of six. It seems likely that the condition has been known before;

see Friedmann, Fraser and Froggatt (1966) for reference to other affected families.

The type of inheritance is discussed in Fraser, Froggatt and Murphy (1964), and the cardiac pathology is fully described in Fraser, Froggatt and James (1964).

The histopathology of the ear has been described for two cases, a 4 year old girl from County Down and a 4 year old boy from Glasgow, by Friedmann et al. (1966).

The middle ear and mastoid processes were normal in two temporal bones, with evidence of inflammatory changes in two.

The utricle and saccule showed atrophic sensory epithelium of the maculae, and globules of periodic-acid-Schiff (PAS)-positive material were present. More PAS-positive material was present in the cristae, in the fibrous stroma beneath the degenerated epithelium.

Within the four cochleae PAS-positive material was found in the stria vascularis, particularly in the apical coil but present in all coils. The organ of Corti showed degenerative changes, and the tectorial membrane was retracted. Reissner's membrane was collapsed and adherent over the remains of the organ of Corti and to the stria vascularis. In case 2 there was granuloma formation in the stria vascularis, with distinct round-celled infiltration.

The seventh and eighth nerves appeared normal, but the number of neurons in the spiral ganglion was greatly reduced.

Cockayne's syndrome This is deafness associated with retinal atrophy and dwarfism. Additionally:

Large hands and feet.
Kyphoscoliosis.
Lack of subcutaneous facial fat.
Prognathism.
Premature senile appearance.
Mental deficiency, commonly microcephalic.
Sensitivity to sunlight, hence pigmentation and scarring.
Cataracts.
Cold blue extremities.
Carious teeth.

All known cases are of Anglo-Saxon descent. Cockayne's syndrome is considered to be inherited by autosomal recessive gene. Paddison *et al.* (1963) found no chromosomal abnormalities in two patients or in their father. They give a detailed account of the post-mortem findings, including the central nervous system. The findings included hydrocephaly, probably secondary to severe cortico-subcentral atrophy. The leptomeninges contained excessive collagenous connective tissue. The cerebral cortex showed evidence of widespread loss of neurons, particularly in the third cortical layers. The calcarine cortex particularly showed leptomeningeal fibrosis, shrunken gyri and reduction of white matter. Widespread dark encrustations were present on numerous cortical capillaries, and in the globus pallidus, and in the media and adventitia of small arterioles. The authors conclude this was a sidero-calcific deposit. In addition, lipofuscin was found in most neurons of the brain stem, but not the cortex.

Ohno and Hirooka (1966) described the findings in renal biopsies in two cases. These were as follows: the glomeruli were 'insufficient in formation', and there was some reduction in the number of capillary loops. The majority of the glomeruli revealed a slight thickening of the mesangium and basement membrane without nuclear proliferation. In some advanced lesions, hyalinisation or collapse was observed. The tubules were sometimes atrophied, with thickening of the basement membrane, and some were dilated, containing protein-like precipitates. Interstitial fibrosis was also found. There was neither cellular infiltration nor arteriosclerotic changes of the vessels, excluding glomerulonephritis, pyelonephritis and nephrosclerosis.

One of their cases was studied for abnormal chromosome development. None was found.

Pendred's syndrome (see also chapter VI) The association of sporadic goitre with congenital deafness is a manifestation of recessive inheritance: as a syndrome it was first described by Pendred in 1896. According to Fraser (1965), the association has been frequently missed owing to the prevalence of endemic goitre.

Brain (1927) reported five east London families, among whom twelve individuals were affected. He postulated that the goitre and the deafness were pleiotropic effects of the same abnormal gene in homozygous form. Brain clearly foreshadowed that the specific inborn failure of metabolism associated with the goitre might be failure to synthesise thyroxine. The subject may be hypothyroid or euthyroid. The type of deafness is perceptive and clinically consistent with a hair-cell lesion.

The histology of the thyroid gland is of over-stimulation by the pituitary so as sometimes to resemble malignancy (Smith, 1960). Smith summarises the thyroid histopathology as nodular, containing colloid, with a highly proliferative epithelium, resulting in papillary formation.

There are four published reports of temporal-bone pathology from cases of deafness and goitre (Fraser *et al.*, 1965). They are: Manasse, P. (1909), *Z. Ohrenheilk.* *58*, 105; Brock, X. (1920), *Arch. Ohrenheilk.* *105*, 135; Nager, F.R. (1925), *Zeit. Hals. Nas. Ohrenheilk.* *11*, 149; Albrecht, W. (1944), *Zeit. Hals. Nas. Ohrenheilk.* *50*, 63. Unfortunately the histological descriptions are inconsistent, and it may be that none was a Pendred's syndrome. Fraser (1964) considered that none was a well documented case of the syndrome.

Hereditary nerve deafness associated with diabetes mellitus has been reported by Hognestad (1967). There appears to be some evidence for considering the family described as showing some relationship of the two diseases: the marriage between a man 'hard of hearing since his thirties' and a woman who 'developed diabetes and reduced hearing in her later years' resulted in twelve children, of whom only two males and one female suffered apparently from neither disease by the age of at least 40 years. The one affected male child had a high-tone hearing loss by middle age—but claimed to have been exposed to a noisy environment (whaling). Three females had both diseases. The other five females had high-tone hearing loss. Most of the third generation is of course too young to have reached the relevant years, but one female had both diseases by 29 years of age. Hognestad considers that the grandfather introduced the gene for hearing loss, the grandmother for diabetes. The progressive perceptive deafness appears to be of dominant inheritance, possibly sex-linked, i.e. in the X-chromosome. Diabetes is usually considered to be of recessive inheritance yet is already present in three generations. It may be that diabetes worsens the nerve deafness, as would be expected if the deafness were an exaggeration of presbyacusis due to arterial disease, for example.

Indeed, two females noted a worsening in their hearing at the time of onset of diabetes.

There is no histopathology of the inner ear in Hognestad's paper.

Three members of the family had urinary tract anomalies and a double uvula. There is no mention of hypertension, nor of the causes of death.

Alstrom *et al.* (1959) describe the syndrome of optic atrophy, nerve deafness, diabetes and obesity.

Usher's syndrome   This is associated with retinitis pigmentosa and perceptive deafness. It is of recessive inheritance, and was first clinically described by von Graefe (1858). The pathology of the membranous cochlea conforms with the Scheibe type, but with widespread involvement of the vestibular apparatus (Siebenmann and Bing, 1907; Nager, 1925).

Doubtful inheritance

A Mondini abnormality, with eosinophilic deposits   The Mondini type of bony cochlear abnormality, regarded by some (see Altmann 1950, 1964) as of dominant inheritance, is thought by Fraser to be of 'unclear' hereditary status. A case is described by Gussen (1968) of a man of 31 years who died with secondaries from carcinoma of colon and sarcoid for which he had been on steroids. He had been deaf from six years of age; his parents and relatives were not deaf, but his parents were uncle and niece.

Genetically, this history is suggestive of a recessive inheritance or of mutation. There is, further, a vague history of trauma at 6 years. The patient's younger only brother, however, developed mild hearing loss mixed in type from 10 years.

The histopathology of the cochlea included:

1. Incomplete separation of the middle and apical cochlear turns.
2. A scala communis in these turns.
3. Reissner's membrane adherent partially to the stria vascularis.
4. No hair-cells present.
5. Wispy tectorial membrane seen in apical turns.
6. Moderate atrophy of the stria vascularis in all turns.
7. A polypoid projection in the middle turn. This was an

elongated cystic structure containing pale eosinophilic granular material probably proteinaceous.

8. Numerous eosinophilic, round or oval hyaline structures were
   present in all turns, abutting on the scala vestibular surface
   of Reissner's membrane. These were covered by flat cells, and
   were strongly PAS-positive.
9. No nerve fibres seen in any laminae.
10. Enormous endolymphatic duct and sac dilatation.
11. Distended saccula, with PAS-positive globules in the maculae
    of both saccule and utricle.

Gussen annotates the occurrence of PAS-positive material in other
recorded cases, and concluded that, in this case, it may be evidence
of previous hydrops, involving the effort of transporting large
volumes of fluid across membranes. No such state had existed in the
cochlear duct, and no PAS-positive material was found there.

The saccule, endolymphatic duct and sac were very dilated, and
contained PAS-positive deposits.

Gussen lists other descriptions of PAS-positive deposits:

1. Friedmann *et al.* (1966) identified such material intravascularly
   in the stria vascularis, and in fibrotic subepithelial tissues beneath the maculae and in the cristae of ampullae in two cases
   of the cardio-auditory syndrome of Jervell and Lange Nielsen.
2. Altmann (1964): globules in the stria vascularis and saccular
   epithelium in a cochleo-saccular type inherited recessive deafness.
3. Buch and Jorgensen (1963): in the epithelial layer of the stria
   vascularis and the saccule and endolymphatic duct of a deaf-
   mute woman, and in a case of Nager's.

Wolff (1949) and Altmann (1950) found hyaline or calcified thrombi
in the stria of deaf-mutes.

*Familial febrile illness, with urticaria and perceptive deafness and
generalised amyloidosis* A Derbyshire family exhibits this syndrome, which is described by Muckle and Wells (1962). Temporal
bones from two of the cases were described by Friedmann (see
Muckle and Wells). The findings were, in a brother and sister,
absence of the organ of Corti and vestibular sensory epithelium,
atrophy of the cochlear nerve, ossification of the basilar membrane,
but no amyloid deposits.

Perceptive deafness occurs rarely with amyloidosis (Chambers *et al.*, 1958).

References

Alport, A.C. (1927), *Brit. Med. Jl. 1,* 504.
Alstrom, C.H., Hallgren, B., Nillson, L.B., and Aglander, H. (1959), *Acta Psychiat. Neurol. Scand. 34*, suppl., 129.
Altmann, F. (1950), *Arch. Otolaryng. 51*, 852.
— (1964), *Acta Otolaryng.*, suppl., 187.
Arnott, E.J., Crawfurd, M.d'A., and Toghill, P.J. (1966), *B. J. Opthal. 50*, 390.
Arthur, L.J.H. (1965), *Devel. Med. Child Neurol. 7*, 395.
Atlee, W.H.W. (1901), *St Barts Hosp. 9*, 41.
Brain, W.R. (1927), *Q. J. Med. 20*, 303.
Buch, N.H., and Jørgensen, M.B. (1963), *Arch. Otolaryng. 77*, 246.
Castleman, B. (1957), *New Eng. J. Med. 257*, 1231.
Chambers, R.A., Medd, W.E., and Spencer, H. (1958), *Q. J. Med. 27*, 207.
Cockayne, E.A. (1936), *Arch. Dis. Child, 11*, 1.
Crawfurd, M. d'A., and Toghill, P.J. (1968), *Q. J. Med. 37*, 516.
Danish, J.M., Tillson, J.K., and Levitan, M. (1963), *Eugenics Q. 10*, 12.
Di George, A.M., Olmstead, R.W., and Harley, R.D. (1960), *J. Pediatr. 57*, 649.
Fisch, L. (1959), *J. Laryng. 73*, 355.
Fraser, G.R., Morgans, M.E., and Trotter, W.R. (1960), *Q. J. Med. 29*, 279.
Fraser, G.R. (1964), *J. Med. Genet, 1*, 118.
— (1965), *Ann. Hum. Genet. 28*, 201.
Fraser, G.R., Froggatt, P., and Murphy, T. (1964), *Ann. Hum. Genet. 28*, 133.
Fraser, G.R., Froggatt, P., and James, T.N. (1964), *Q. J. Med. 33*, 361.
Friedmann, I., Fraser, G.R., and Froggatt, P. (1966), *J. Laryng. 80*, 451.
Gardner, W.J., and Turner, O. (1940), *Arch. Neurol. Psychiatr. 44*, 76.
Gates, R.R. (1946), *Human Genetics*, Macmillan, New York.
Goldbloom, R.B., Fraser, F.C., Waugh, G., Aronovitch, M., and Wiglesworth, F.W. (1957), *Pediatrics, 20*, 241.
Gregg, J.B., and Becker, S.F. (1963), *Arch. Ophthal.* (Chicago), *69*, 293.
Gussen, R. (1968), *J. Laryng. 82*, 41.
Hamburger, J., Crosnier, J., Lissal, J., and Naffal, J. (1956), *J. Urol. 62*, 113.

Hognestad, S. (1967), *Acta Otolaryng. 64*, 219.
Krickstein, H.I., Gloor, G.J., and Balogh, K. (1966), *Arch. Path. 82*, 506.
McDonald, R., and Harrison, V.C. (1965), *Ann. Pediatr. 4*, 739.
Muckle, T.J., and Wells, M. (1962), *Q. J. Med. 31*, 235.
Nager, F.R. (1925), *Z. Hals. Nas. Ohr. 11*, 149.
Ohno, T., and Hirooka, M. (1966), *Tohoku J. Exp. Med. 89*, 151.
Paddison, R.M., Moossy, J., Derbes, V.J., and Kiloepferber (1963), *Derm. Trop. 2*, 195.
Pendred, V. (1896), *Lancet, 2*, 532.
Perkoff, G.T., Nugent, G.A., Dolowitz, D.A., Stephens, F.E., Carnes, W.H., and Tyler, F.H. (1958), *A.M.A. Arch. Int. Med. 102*, 733.
Robin, E.D., Gardner, F.H., and Levine, S.A. (1957), *Trans. Assn. Amer. Phys. 70*, 140.
Rosen, S., Pirani, C.L., and Muehrcke, R.C. (1966), *Am. J. Clin. Path. 45*, 32.
Siebenmann, F., and Bing, R. (1907), *Z. Ohrenheilk. 54*, 265.
Smith, J.F. (1960), *Q. J. Med. 29*, 297.
Sohar, E. (1956), *A.M.A. Arch. Int. Med. 97*, 627.
— (1954), *Harefuah, 27*, 161.
Usher, C.H. (1914), *Roy. Lond. Ophthal. Hosp. Rep. 19*, 130.
Von Graefe, A. (1858), *Arch. Ophthal. 4*, 250.
Wallace, I.R., and Jones, J.H. (1960), *Lancet, 1*, 941.
Williamson, D.A.J. (1961), *Lancet, 2*, 1321.
Wildervanck, L.S. (1963), *Acta Genet.*, Basel, *13*, 161.
Wolff, D. (1949), *Trans. Amer. Acad. Ophth. Otolaryng. 54*, 37.
Waardenburg, P.J. (1951), *J. Hum. Genet. 3*, 195.

IX Hereditary disorders of connective tissue; the mucopolysaccharidoses

Hürler's syndrome, Hunter–Hürler's syndrome, etc.

This is a rare inherited disorder, probably autosomal-recessive, and commoner in males. Clinically, there is dwarfing, grotesque bodily formation, mental defect and deafness: Hunter and Hürler described it independently. It is a disorder resulting in accumulation of mucopolysaccharide and probably lipids in histiocytes, polymorphonuclear leucocytes and other cells in affected organs, and spilling over into the urine. It is also known as gargoylism, Hürler–Pfaundler syndrome, lipochondrodystrophy or dysostosis multiplex.

Differential diagnosis

1. *Cretinism.* In Hürler's disease the bone age is normal, and the thyroid function also; the patient is active.

2. *Congenital syphilis.* Hürler's disease is not primarily periostitis, and the deformities in the spine are due to abnormal discs and ligaments. Nor is 'serology' positive in Hürler's disease.

Rapid clinical diagnosis. A filter-paper test exists, which depends on a change of colour of dried urine in filter paper when acetic acid and toluidine blue are added. The mucopolysaccharide is metachromatic, so the blueness becomes pink and purple if it is present.

Rapid diagnostic tests. Muir's method for cytology of blood films for lymphocytic granules; for these, toluidine blue is specific, May–Gruenwald is not.

Pathology Cartilage, ligaments, tendons and cornea are involved. Large, clear, vacuolated gargoyle cells are present, and clusters of swollen collagen fibres. Liver-cell disturbance may lead to fibrosis and portal hypertension. Aortic valve disease may result in cardiac ischaemia, which may also be caused by occlusion of a coronary artery by deposits of gargoyle cells in the intima.

Dawson (1954) considered the substance polysaccharide or muco-polysaccharide. In the neurones and parenchymal cells, deposits include phosphates and cerebrosides, which is suggestive of a meta-chromatic leucodystrophy. Meyer (1961) has identified heparitin, a highly branched mucopolysaccharide. For distinctions between the different types of mucopolysaccharidosis, see tables v and vii.

Table V Six forms of genetic mucopolysaccharidosis, I–VI (McKusick *et al.*, 1965)

Syndrome	Remarks	Mucopolysaccharide(s) involved
I. Hürler syndrome	Early corneal clouding. Hepatosplenomegaly and retinal degeneration. Grave manifestations, mental and somatic, early death. Coronary occlusions, aortic valves.	Chondroitin sulphate B and heparatin sulphate.
II. Hunter syndrome	No clouding of cornea. Milder course than Hürler's.	Chondroitin sulphate B
III. Sanfilippo syndrome	Mild somatic. Late onset, retarding mentally. Severe CNS effects.	Heparatin sulphate
IV. Morquio syndrome	Severe bone change. Cloudy cornea, visceral effects and in urine. Intellect may be affected. Aortic regurgitation.	Kerato-sulphate
V. Scheie syndrome	Stiff joints. Cloudy cornea. Coarse facies. Aortic regurgitation.	Chondroitin sulphate B
VI. Maroteaux–Lamy syndrome	Striking skeletal changes. Unimpaired intelligence.	Chondroitin sulphate B

All are autosomal recessive, except II, which is X-linked recessive. Deafness has been reported in types I and II only.

Nelson (1964) leaves the aetiology of deafness unconsidered, though he mentions nasopharyngeal scarring, which might imply middle-ear disease, and Eustachian obstruction, especially in con-junction with reduced ability to withstand infections.

6—P.D.

Table VI Mucopolysaccharides

Non-sulphated MPS	Hexosamine	Hexuronic acid	Normal location
Chondroitin	Galactosamine	Glucuronic	Cornea and vitreous
Hyaluronic acid	Glucosamine	Glucuronic	Synovial fluid
Sulphated MPS			
Ketarosulphate	Glucosamine Galactose	None	Cornea Cartilage Nucleus pulposus
Heparitin sulphate	Glucosamine	Glucuronic	Aorta
Chondroitin sulphate A	Galactosamine	Glucuronic	Cornea Cartilage
Chondroitin sulphate B	Galactosamine	Iduronic	Skin Heart Aorta
Chondroitin sulphate C	Galactosamine	Glucuronic	Cartilage Tendon
Heparin	Glucosamine	Glucuronic	Liver Mast cells

Table VII Fuller clinical descriptions of all types

Deafness is described in types I and II only.

I. *McKusick et al.'s two brothers with Hürler's syndrome.*

Both were deaf but had no history of otitis media.
Saddle nose and typical Hürler faces.
Short stumpy broad phalanges and metacarpals.
Oedema of eyelids.
Wide-spaced teeth.
Corneal opacity.
Low-set ears.
Lumbar gibbus.
Stiff joints.
Hepatosplenomegaly.
Inguinal hernias.
Urine positive, lymphocytes 10–18 per cent positive, for mucopolysaccharide.

II. *The Hunter syndrome*

Progressive deafness of a perceptive type since 7 years old.
No lumbar gibbus.
Face of a plethoric farmer.
No pectus excavatus.
No clinical corneal opacity; but it may be seen with slit-lamp.
Adult life possible (33 years).
One case reads the *Wall Street Journal.*
Knock knees.
Hepatosplenomegaly.

Cardiac enlargement.

No family history, as often happens where X-linked-affected males do not reproduce.

Urine positive, lymphocytes 20 per cent positive for mucopolysaccharide.

III. *Sanfilippo type*

Deafness not reported here.

No clinical corneal clouding.

Dwarfing and joint stiffness and hepatosplenomegaly moderate.

Not usually weak, but severe mental changes come on during childhood and adolescence. Speech deteriorating by 8 years.

Coarse Hürler features, short neck.

Normal height. But by 12 years stopped talking and was incontinent.

Clubbing of fingers by puberty at 15.

First teeth normal, second were wide and small.

Thickened calvarium.

Urine positive, lymphocytes positive 20 per cent and 28 per cent in brother and a sister who was also affected. Two other unrelated cases showed 40 per cent and 60 per cent positive lymphocytes.

IV. *Morquio–Brailsford type*

(Possibly reported by Osler, and Voisin and Voisin as achondroplasias.) Others reported as Morquio's disease are possibly not rightly classified (*McKusick*).

No mention is made of deafness.

If these cases with skeletal abnormalities live to adolescence, they develop corneal or ocular lesions, and usually cardiac.

Rather similar skeletal changes to Hürler type, leading to a semi-crouching position, but the vertebrae are flat and thinned.

Corneal hazing is present, and there may be granularity of the macula. The cause of death is cardiac failure.

Reilly bodies are present in the leucocytes, the majority of the polymorpho-nuclears. No granules can be detected in the lymphocytes, but the urine is positive for mucopolysaccharide.

V. *Scheibe type*

No impairment of intellect: some 'near genius'.

Hearing was reported as deteriorating at 46 in one case, one ear, probably cochlea is location of lesion. Marked clouding of cornea is present, and aortic stenosis.

One case showed 1–3 per cent lymphocytes positive, and one negative for metachromatic granules. The macrophages may be positive, however.

Urine is usually positive for mucopolysaccharide.

VI. *Maroteaux–Lamy type*

This type exhibits striking osseous changes, as bad as I or II, but no mental impairment, and no deafness.

Chondroitin sulphate B is present in urine, lymphocytes and in polymorphs.

Pathology of deafness in this condition. Kelemen (1966) has described the histological findings in two cases (*q.v. infra.*) and refers to three other reports in which histology findings are presented (Wolff, 1942; De Lange *et al.*, 1944; Ricci and Ancetti, 1955). In a clinical report Kittel (1963) tabulated seventy-eight cases, of which 28 per cent were hard of hearing or totally deaf. It is clear from McKusick *et al.* (1965) that there are six clinically similar but fundamentally distinct forms of abnormal mucopolysaccharidoses. These are genetic in origin: all are autosomal recessive, apart from Hunter's, which appears to be X-linked. Unfortunately no clear correlation with deafness is described, nor do we easily classify those cases with cochlear histology mentioned in Kelemen's paper. But the normal distribution of these mucopolysaccharides, which are hexosamines conjugated with hexuronic acids, may assist in this: table vi summarises the distribution. Deafness is accordingly accepted in i (Hürler) and ii (Hunter). Kelemen's cases are almost certainly Hürler's or type i, with early death. Both were males and died at 3 or 4 years respectively. The histological findings were as follows.

Both temporal bones showed a 'high papillomatous mucous membrane, with comparative scarcity of vessels'. The mucosa blocked the oval and the round window niches. In one case persistent mesenchyme extended from the pneumatic system well into the tympanic cavity, including the epitympanum where it tightly surrounded the ossicles. Kelemen considered that signs of chronic ear infection in such young patients indicated an intra-uterine origin of the inflammatory process, but the relevance of this is doubtful.

Case i showed the pneumatic cells filled with persistent mesenchyme, and the middle ear filled with high mucous membrane, containing cysts. The end of the long process of the incus was destroyed. An osteoma-like inclusion was found near the round window, and one in the niche of the round window, and another arose nearby on a slender pedicle. The spiral ligament showed some calcification.

Case 2 had hardly any middle ear lumen: the inner ear was preserved and showed calcification of the spiral ligament on the basal turn, as in case i; the organ of Corti was depressed but its elements were discernible. Reissner's membrane was straight in section. The modiolar canal was well filled. The maculae and cristae were normal. The cochlear wall of the basal turn showed a large resorption area penetrating two layers, but leaving the endosteum intact. It was composed of large, clear cells, with peripherally placed nuclei; these Kelemen considered were 'gargoyle cells', vacuolised chondrocytes as described by McKusick (1960). The appearances are not completely convincing from the photomicrograph.

There would have been added complications in the way of infections, but Kelemen concludes that the persistent mesenchyme, the reduced middle-ear cavity and the filled windows are sufficient to cause the deafness.

If there is calcification of the spiral ligament, it is probable that there are ground-substance disturbances there.

De Lange *et al.* (1944) describe the case of a boy of 19 who had had skeletal deformity and some mental retardation, incontinence at 6 years, and severe deafness of a perceptive kind. There was a history of otitis media as well. At post-mortem thickened connective tissue was found in the trachea and larynx as had been during life: the appearances were that of a chondroid or a mucoid alteration of the connective tissue. The petrous temporal bones showed incomplete pneumatisation of the mastoid process, with a fibrous mucous membrane. There was a focus of otosclerosis in the otic capsule beneath the basal turn. The scala vestibuli and scala tympani were normal. The ductus cochleae was partly collapsed. The organ of Corti was a heap of undifferentiated cells. The ganglion spirale in the basal turn showed few ganglion cells, and lymphocyte infiltration. There was a marked mucoid degeneration of connective tissues of various parts of the body. The brain was normal. (Papers not illustrated.)

Ricci and Ancetti (1955) described the petrous bone in a child of 7 years. Their paper is well illustrated. The main changes are collapse of Reissner's membrane; in the otic capsule there are numerous cartilaginous rests, not unlike an otosclerotic focus in some ways. The cochlear canal appears to contain a deposit, and the lining of the scala vestibuli and scala tympani is covered under a thicker layer of an eosinophilic deposit which may be suggestive of an earlier infection involving the cochlea. The organ of Corti is degenerate. The stria vascularis is possibly normal. The ganglion cells show a reduction in numbers.

Wolff describes one case (1942) with small mastoid antra, porous bone and irregular areas of dense fibrosis with irregular calcium deposits. Some exudate was found in the middle ear. Irregular contours of the semi-circular canals were found. Within one round window irregular bony nodules protruded into the scala tympani. Reissner's membrane was 'intact'. The spiral ligament contained large cystic spaces surrounded by dense fibrosis. The stria vascularis had disintegrated. Rosenthal's canal was devoid of nerve fibres. Spiral ganglion cells stained faintly and showed vacuolated cytoplasm, though not appreciably decreased in number.

It remains for a pathologist interested in these conditions to obtain a temporal bone suitably fixed for a study of mucopolysaccharides (Poulsen, 1966), which may be more important within the cochlea and middle ear than is shown by these reports. Although Pearse (1961) states that formalin with or without mercury is an adequate fixative for mucopolysaccharides, material that has to be decalcified may require other treatment, such as lead acetate followed by EDTA decalcification.

Austin et al. (1964) have shown that arylsulphatase-B activity is increased in 'gargoylism'. It is a lysosomal enzyme, as are acid phosphatase, β-galactosidase and arylsulphatase-A. Studied by workers in 'gargoylism' and in metachromatic leucodystrophy, this is another genetically controlled 'storage' disease, where accumulations of cerebroside sulphatides are found in the nervous system and the kidney. Arylsulphatase-A was low in metachromatic leucodystrophy disease, and as the β-galactosidase and the acid phosphatase of the lysosomes were normal, these authors found it difficult to attribute the low sulphatase activities to a secondary non-specific degeneration of lysosomes, i.e. caused by damage to cells by the accumulations. The 'gargoyle' children had high arylsulphatase-B activity in the white matter, the liver and the kidney.

The interest of this group of diseases lies in their similarity in some ways to otosclerosis, which is also genetically controlled, though dominant. It is also a disease affecting bone and soft tissue growth in or near the otic capsule. The deafness comes on in young adult life in otosclerosis rather than in childhood, and as far as is known the otosclerotic changes are not manifest elsewhere in the skeleton.

References

Austin, J., McAfee, D., Armstrong, D., O'Rourke, M., Shearer, L., and Bachhaivat, B. (1964), *Biochem. J. 93*, 15.

Dawson, I.M.P. (1954) *J. Path. Bact. 67*, 587.

De Lange, C., Gerlings, P.G., de Kleyn, A., and de Lettinga, T.W. (1944), *Acta Paediatr. 31*, 398.

Gardner, D.L. (1965), *Pathology of the Connective Tissue Diseases,* Arnold, London.

Hunter, C. (1916–17), *Proc. Roy. Soc. Med. 10*, 104.

Hürler, G. (1919), *Z. Kinderheilk. 24*, 220.

Kelemen, G. (1966), *Z. Laryng. Rhin. 80*, 791.

Kittel, G. (1963), *Z. Laryng. Rhin. 42*, 206.

Leroy, J.G., and Crocker, A.C. (1966), *A. J. Dis. Child, 112*, 518.

McKusick, V.A. (1960), *Heritable Disorders of Connective Tissue,* second edition, St Louis, Mo.

McKusick, V.A., Kaplan, D., Wise, D., Hanley, W.B., Suddarth, S.B., Sevick, S.B., and Maumenee, A.E. (1965), *Medicine* (Baltimore), *44*, 445.

Meyer (1961), see Gardner (1965).

Muir, H., Mittwoch, V., and Bitter, T. (1963), *Arch. Dis. Child, 38*, 358.

Nelson, W.E. (1964), *Textbook of Pediatrics*, eighth edition, Saunders, Philadelphia, Pa.

Pearse, A.G.E. (1961), *Histochemistry*, second edition, Churchill.

Poulsen, H. (1966) in *Hormones and Connective Tissue*, ed. G. Ashoe-Hansen, Munksgaard, Copenhagen.

Ricci, V., and Ancetti, A. (1955), *Arch. Ital. Otol. 66*, 734.

Wolff, D. (1942), *Laryngoscope, 52*, 218.

X The collagen diseases

Myositis ossificans progressiva

Three of Lutwak's six cases (1964) of this disease were partially deaf; although he identified 258 cases of the disease within world literature he does not detail deafness. All of his three patients were female. The 34 year old was described as suffering from a bilateral nerve deafness, the other two, 23 and 31, showed decreased air-conduction only. Ludman *et al.* (1968) report three cases with deafness, and discuss the possible causation of the deafness. One patient was male, whose hearing was a low-tone conductive deafness by 18 years of age. The other two, whose deafness came on in childhood soon after the general disease was diagnosed, were also 'conductive' in type. These two also had microdactyly of the big toes, often associated with the generalised disease. It is possible that the deafness is due to stapedius ossification, or to otosclerosis, or it may be coincidental.

No pathology of the disease appears in the literature. McKusick (1960) regards the disease as due to a dominant gene with reduced penetrance.

Cogan's syndrome

Cogan (1945) described a case of perceptive deafness associated with non-syphilitic interstitial keratitis. By 1965 Wolff *et al.* had seen reports of thirty-six cases, and reported one of their own, in which post-mortem examination had been made and the temporal bones examined microscopically. Only one other such case was known (Fischer and Hellstrom, 1961). Both cases showed new bone formation within the scala tympani, destruction of the tectorial membrane, and dilatation of the scala media.

The aetiology remains obscure: some cases have been associated with polyarteritis nodosa, others with virus diseases.

Lindsay (1965, in discussion after Wolff *et al.*'s paper describing the pathology of the second case of Cogan's syndrome) suggests that there is a possibility of invasion of the labyrinth from the cochlear aqueducts by some inflammatory process, and quotes a case of Nager's (1907), of meningo-encephalitis following measles, in which a similar histological picture of new bone formation in the scala tympani was found. He also had a case. There is a similar case at the Institute of Laryngology and Otology.

Wolff *et al.*'s findings (well illustrated) were as follows. There was much 'blue mantling' in the otic capsule, and new bone formation in the region of the round window, occupying much of the scala tympani of the basal coil of the cochlea, and the perilymphatic space of the distal curve of the posterior semi-circular canal. Excess fluid was present in the scala media and there was 'hypertrophy' of the stria vascularis. Reissner's membrane had ruptured in places. A cyst was seen in the stria of the middle turn. The organ of Corti was least degenerated in this turn. The tectorial membrane was not present in any coil. There were oedema of the spiral ligament, and the appearances of invasion by the epithelial cells of the stria. In addition, there was atrophy of spiral ganglion cells in the middle turns at least. There was also a delicate areolar connective tissue in much of the scala tympani and scala vestibuli, possibly an antecedent of bone.

This case died following a hemiparesis: the pathologist's 'closing observation' was that all the patient's disabling disorders had followed a mild or severe infection during the first week or two of recovery, and suggested an autogenous sensitivity. There is no record suggestive of autoimmune disorder in this case.

Serrins *et al.* (1963), however, recall that cases may be associated with eosinophilia as high as 28 per cent. They review the literature and conclude that the disease belongs in the 'collagen' group. There is no mention of tests for 'autoimmune' disorders such as rheumatoid factor, antinuclear factor, thydroid precipitins.

With the similarity to late-onset deafness in congenital syphilis, both in the accompanying interstitial keratitis and of the evidence of new bone formation within the labyrinth, the absence of recorded results of specific treponemal serology is to be deplored. It is certainly possible that Cogan's syndrome is, after all, syphilitic but with negative STS (standard tests for syphilis).

The case reported by Cogan and Dickersin (1964) was found to have patchy infiltration by polymorphonuclears and lymphocytes in the aortic intima. This was a boy of 14 years of age, with a polymorphonuclear leucocytosis and normal CSF findings. These authors found no evidence of polyarteritis nodosa, as had been found in three previous autopsies (Crawford, 1957; Eisenstein and Taubenhaus, 1958; Fischer and Hellstrom, 1962). Cogan's and Dickersin's case died of congestive cardiac failure following a long illness beginning with granular opacities in the cornea and deafness, followed by anaemia, aortic regurgitation and renal failure. The aorta contained large mural thrombi in the thoracic and abdominal portions. The Hinton test (a screening test for lues) had been negative in the patient and his parents: this would hardly have been so in a juvenile syphilitic aortitis.

This case lends support to the 'collagen' disease theory of the aetiology of Cogan's disease.

Rheumatoid arthritis

Copeman (1963) described three cases of deafness which appeared to have strong associations with rheumatoid arthritis, and suggested that as these were conductive in type, and improved as the arthritis improved, the cause was an exudate in the synovial joints of the ossicular chains. Ransome (1964) agreed that as rheumatoid arthritis had been long known to affect the crico-arytenoid joints there was no reason why other synovial joints should not be affected, and mentioned two cases of rheumatoid arthritis of long standing in which unilateral permanent conductive deafness was found which did not fit a diagnosis of otosclerosis clinically. She further mentions the possibility of deafness during exacerbations due to salicylate poisoning (Covell, 1936).

Arslan (1963), in a review of collagen disease of the ear, nose and throat, does not mention such a form of deafness.

One temporal bone of a rheumatoid patient was examined, unfortunately from a case with clinically normal hearing, and no abnormality was found by the author.

References

Arslan, M. (1963), *Acta Otolaryng., supp. 183*, 14.
Cogan, D.G. (1945), *Arch. Ophthal. 33*, 144.
Cogan, D.G., and Dickersin, C.R. (1964), *Arch. Ophthal. 74*, 80.
Copeman, W.S.C. (1963), *Brit. Med. Jl. 2*, 1526.
Covell, W.P. (1936), *Arch. Otolaryng. 23*, 633.
Crawford (1957), see Cogan and Dickersin (1964).
Eisenstein and Taubenhaus, see Cogan and Dickersin (1964).
Fisher, E.R., and Hellstrom, H.R. (1961), *Arch. Path. 72*, 572.
Lindsay, J.R. (1965), *Trans. Amer. Otol. Soc. 53*, 108.
Ludman, H., Hamilton, E.B.D., and Eade, A.W.T. (1968), *J. Laryng. 82*, 57.
Lutwak, L. (1964), *Amer. J. Med. 37*, 269.
McKusick, V.A. (1960), *Heritable Disorders of Connective Tissue*, second edition, St Louis, Mo.
Ransome, J. (1964), *Brit. Med. Jl. 1*, 179.
Serrins, A.J., Harrison, R., and Chandler, J.R. (1963), *Arch. Otolaryng. 78*, 785.
Wolff, D., Bernhardt, W.G., Tsutsumi, S., Ross, T., and Nussbaum, N.E. (1965), *Trans. Amer. Otol. Soc. 53*, 94.

XI Otosclerosis

This is a difficult disease to classify pathologically. It is the commonest cause of adult deafness, and it may be accepted as a disease of bone, or at least within bone, in a minutely localised area. Clinically, deafness is due to fixation by ossification of the stapes within the oval window. There may be a lesion of the whole or part of the stapes and different parts of the otic capsule. If a lesion is found which does not affect the stapedial joint-space, conductive deafness is unlikely. The term otosclerosis presumably refers to the rigidity of the stapes, for the histological picture of the lesion is not sclerotic but extremely vascular, and may contain marrow spaces. New bone formation is evident, and it is woven bone which differs from the normal lamellar bone. Such a process may become inactive, or may progress. The vascular walls and ground substance stain intensively, and are deeply basophilic on haematoxylin and eosin staining ('blue mantles'). The number of osteoblasts is increased in an active lesion. A small lesion may suggest that primarily this indeed might be vascular because of the much-branded appearance of the vessels.

The histological appearances are those of new bone, with a web-like collagen pattern. The collagen has a normal periodicity, that is, bands at 640 Å, and may be considered normal. The lesion progresses to considerable increase in size and deformity of the stapes. There is no convincing evidence as to the initiation of new bone growth.

Cinca of Bucharest has calculated that there are at least sixty-two theories of the aetiology of this disease, according to Chevance (1969), who considers that only a study of the cytology and ultrastructure of the diseased cells can contribute to useful knowledge.

It has been found that a survey of human temporal bones will yield about ten per cent with signs of otosclerosis, but only one per cent in a site which affects hearing (Engström, 1939; Guild, 1944;

Jorgensen and Kristensen, 1967). Morrison (1967) estimated that the incidence of deafness from this condition in an east London population was three per 1,000, but that the frequency of histological otosclerosis was seven per 1,000.

Whatever the initial pathology, there is little doubt that there is good evidence for inheritance as a dominant gene which may lead in adult life to a histological lesion. If the site is appropriate, there will be deafness. No correlation was found by Morrison with ABO, MN or Rh blood groups, or secretor status, or the haptoglobin genotypes.

Chromosome studies have shown that the carriers of the gene (genotypes) and sufferers from the disease (phenotypes) were normal karyotypes. The suggestion of Tato et al. (1963) that trisomy 13 might be responsible, with mosaicism of forty-six, forty-seven or forty-eight chromosomes, has not been confirmed.

Apart from chromosomal abnormalities, the following have been noted as having some bearing on aetiology:

1. *Change in enzymatic activity of osteocytes* (Chevance, 1964). The changes of appearance and number of osteocytes may be those of normal growing bone, but acid mucopolysaccharide increases as well as alkaline phosphatase activity. (Wullstein et al. (1960) observed alkaline phosphatase in the endolymph of otosclerotic patients.)

2. *Metabolic functions*, such as the 30 per cent higher lactic dehydrogenase activity of vein tissue found in otosclerotics (Soifer et al., 1965). Vyslonzil (1956), Bentzen (1961) and Stadil (1961) have reported mucopolysaccharide accumulation in the skin of otosclerotics when compared with normal people of the same age group.

3. *Endocrine*. The disease has long been considered to deteriorate during pregnancy and lactation (Cawthorne, 1955). The identification of a significant number of otosclerotics in a series of acromegalics is interesting (Richards, 1968).

4. *Factors concerned in promoting bone growth* might account for the worsening or onset of a similar lesion, in the course of healing of fractures of osteogenesis imperfecta.

5. *Factors concerned in undue bone resorption as a precipitation of the lesion* have been considered by Gussen (1967). The role of the globuli interossei, which have the appearances of calcified chondro-

cytes and are usually agreed to be calcified cartilage remnants in enchondral bone, was considered to be in normal bone remodelling. Findings from patients who had been on steroids for several months showed bone resorption in areas of polymerised mucopolysaccharide. These findings are in agreement with Albernaz and Covell (1961), Arslan and Ricci (1963), and Hopp and Burn (1958), confirming the potential importance of ground substance.

6. *Venous shunts between the otosclerotic focus and the capillaries of the stria vascularis.* Rüedi (1965) describes such lesions, accompanied by swollen striae. He postulates that the actively growing otosclerotic lesion thromboses the vessels in the normal bone as it advances, and a connection between the old and the new becomes possible by new arterial capillaries which drain into the old venules of the otic capsule. It follows that once shunts have developed in this way, and as the focus advances, similar shunts might develop between it and the vessels of the mucosa (the flamingo flush of Schwartze) or of the spiral ligament.

Rüedi considers that such shunts could account for the sensori-neural deafness found in some otosclerotics and (1968) in that of Paget's disease and Recklinghausen's disease. It is difficult, however, to accept a histological appearance which is apparently rare as evidence of aetiology of a not uncommon lesion. Further, the age ranges of the patients and the predominance of the basal part of the otic capsule make it essential that the arteriolosclerosis of the stria and the neuronal degeneration of middle and old age should be considered.

7. *The special anatomical location of the fissular regions* (Anson, 1968), because it is the site of predilection. There is little doubt that polymerisation of the mucopolysaccharide may affect both bone resorption and growth, as heparin has been shown to do (Petrovic and Shambaugh, 1968; Goldhaber, 1965), possibly acting as a co-factor. Mucopolysaccharides, a group which chemically includes heparin, are responsible for ion exchange and transport of substances in the tissues; water-holders, and with viscosity affected by hormones, these might thus be expected to maintain normal metabolism of local tissues. If changed in character, adverse or changed metabolism would be expected. They may be produced in vessels of most calibres, and with increase in age may accumulate in the medial coat.

Otosclerosis may be closely bound up with local vascular disturbance, as it sometimes appears to be microscopically. What is far from clear is why hereditary disease should manifest itself so relatively late in life. It may well bear further comparison with the pathology of 'clubbing' (see Bigler, 1958), in which the soft tissues of the nail-bed are thickened, containing new blood vessels, even glomus formations, and an increase in mucopolysaccharides. The lesion can produce new periosteal bone. Fibroblasts are increased. Unlike otosclerosis, perivascular aggregations of lymphocytes are seen, however.

Alternatively, otosclerosis may be an inherited bone dystrophy, with inevitable renewal of bone growth. It occurs in an area of unique bone remodelling before birth (Bast and Anson).

References

Albernaz, P.E.M., and Covell, W.P. (1961), *Laryngoscope, 71,* 1333.

Arslan, M., and Ricci, V. (1963), *J. Laryng. 77,* 365.

Bast, T.H., and Anson, J.B. (1949), *The Temporal Bone and the Ear,* Thomas, Springfield, Ill.

Bentzen, O. (1961), Seventh International Congress of Otolaryngology, Paris. Excerpt in *Med. Abstr.* (Int. Congr. Scr. *35*), Abst. 80.

Bigler, F.C. (1958), *Am. J. Path. 34,* 237.

Cawthorne, T. (1955), *J. Laryng, 69,* 437.

Chevance, L. (1964), *Acta Otolaryng. 58,* 175.

Engström, H. (1939), *Acta Otolaryng. 27,* 608.

Goldhaber, P. (1965), *Science, 147,* 407.

Guild, S. (1944), *Ann. Otol, 53,* 246.

Gussen, R. (1967), *Acta Otolaryng. 63,* 411.

Hopp, E.S., and Burn, H.F. (1958), *Ann. Otol. 67,* 480.

Jorgensen, M.B., and Kristensen, H.K. (1967), *Ann. Otol. 76,* 83.

Morrison, A.W. (1967), *Ann. Roy. Coll. Surg. 41,* 202.

Petrovic, A., and Shambaugh, C.E., Jr. (1968), *Acta Otolaryng. 65,* 120.

Richards, S. (1968), *J. Laryng. 82,* 1053.

Rüedi, L. (1965), *Laryngoscope, 75,* 1582.

— (1966), *Arch. Otolaryng. 83,* 507.

— (1968), *Acta Otolaryng. 65,* 13.

Soifer, N., Altman, F., Endahl, G., and Holdsworth, C.E. (1965), *Arch. Otolaryng. 82,* 510.

Stadil, E. (1961), Seventh International Congress of Otolaryngology, Paris. Excerpt in *Med. Abstr.* (Int. Congr. Ser. *35*), Abst. 331.

Tato, J.M., Valencia, H., and Lozzio, C.B. (1963), *Acta Otolaryng. 56*, 265.

Vyslonzil, E. (1956), *Z. Laryng. Rhin. Otol. 35*, 185.

Wullstein, H.L., Kley, W., Rauch, S., and Köstlin, A. (1960), *Z. f. Laryng. 39*, 665.

XII Disorders of nutrition

Malabsorption

Deafness in children is occasionally associated with:

(*a*) Maternal nutritional deficiency due to the malabsorption syndrome in the mother (Whetnall, 1964).

(*b*) Malabsorption in the child (Whetnall, personal communication, 1963).

The pathology of malabsorption is one of chronic diarrhoea, and resultant loss of nutritional substances, whether by actual inability of the intestine to absorb them, as in the case of fats in chronic pancreatic insufficiency, or of failure of intestinal enzymes to break down sugars to an absorbable form, or by 'intestinal hurry' which appears to reduce the chances of absorption of certain substances such as iron and the water-soluble vitamins. Fat-soluble vitamins will also tend to be lost in those diseases accompanied by steatorrhea.

The main nutrients lost may include:

Fats.
Carbohydrates; disaccharides and monosaccharides may be involved.
Proteins.
Vitamins, including folic acid.
Minerals: calcium, iron, phosphate.

Disaccharides and monosaccharides are normally absorbed into mucosal cells and there the disaccharides are split: for example lactose is split by lactase (β-galactosidase) into glucose and galactose and is thus absorbed into the circulation. A child may have a genetically determined inability to absorb lactose, which results in a fermentative diarrhoea, and an adult may lose the ability to absorb lactose, with the same results.

7—P.D.

Fibrocystic disease of the pancreas   Probably due to a recessive
gene, not very rare among the population. Its occurrence is one in
1,000 live births.

Disaccharide intolerances   Due to lack of intestinal enzymes. These
may be inborn or acquired in later life.

The results vary with the amount of intestinal hurry resulting
from absence of specific enzymes, and may include failure to
absorb fat-soluble vitamins, minerals such as calcium and iron, and
other essentials such as folic acid.

Material from infants affected by these diseases has been examined.
No structural deformity of the cochlea or middle ear was found,
but out of seven cases involving poor nutrition only three had a
completely normal middle ear, and possibly four a normal cochlea.
These included one frank purulent acute otitis, two early exudates,
and one giant-cell exudate. One cochlea had bilateral cochleo-
saccular degeneration, with thin fibrin threads in the scala tympani,
and reduced ganglion cells. Two others showed evidence of infection, and one of the 'normals' had reduced myelinated fibres in the
basal turn. None of the temporal bones received came from a case
of maternal malabsorption, which Whetnall (1964) suggests may
be a cause of congenital deafness.

Inadequate dietary intake, avitaminoses

Vitamin A deficiency   Mellanby (1938) described the experimental
production of deafness in young animals by diet deficient in vitamin
A and carotene, and with excessive cereal. Particularly striking
changes were observed in the labyrinthine capsule and both parts
of the eighth nerve itself. The cochlear branch was more affected
than the vestibular. Mellanby's summary of the results is as follows:

1. The labyrinthine capsules:
   (*a*) Degeneration of different degrees up to complete disappear-
        ance of the cochlear nerve, the cells of the spiral ganglion
        and their central and peripheral branches.
   (*b*) Degeneration, but to a lesser degree, of the vestibular
        division of the eighth nerve.
   (*c*) Overgrowth of bone in the modiolus and of the periosteal
        layer of the capsule near the brain.

2. This overgrowth is apparently responsible for the degenerative changes in the nerves by reason of the compressing and stretching of these tissues.

3. Serous labyrinthitis also develops in the cochlea of dogs on a vitamin A deficient diet. This condition seems to produce degeneration of the sensory epithelium of the labyrinth including that of the organ of Corti and of the ampullae of the semi-circular canals in the course of time.

4. Substitution of potato for the cereal element of these vitamin A deficient diets greatly reduces the abnormal changes in the labyrinth (this implies that vitamin C plays some part).

5. Examination of the base of the skull of these vitamin A deficient dogs reveals other bone overgrowths and deformity, which is probably responsible for the degenerative changes of other cranial nerves, such as the optic and trigeminal.

Perlman (1944), however, considered that this was unlikely to have significance in the human, and refers to a paper—'Uber Exostosen im Porus acusticus internus'—by Manasse containing the only descriptions that resemble the experimental lesion.

Manasse's case is described (in Perlman and Willard, 1941) as an 83 year old man with symmetrical hyperplasia of the base of the skull and internal auditory meatus. There was no involvement of the middle ear aspect of the otic capsule, nor of the bone of the rest of the middle or outer ear. No audiological or histological description is included.

Perlman and Willard (1941) had confirmed in the rabbit the bony hyperplasia of the vitamin A deficient dog. Loch (1939) and Covell (1940) had confirmed these results in the rat. Perlman and Willard found bony changes, which resulted in compression and stretching of the eighth nerve in the internal auditory meatus, but little evidence of cochlear functional deficiency. Perlman (1944) points out that such a condition is unlikely in the human, where vitamin A deficiency is not likely to arise because of large reserves in the liver, and notes that the only reports on death with evidence such as xerophthalmia of human vitamin A deficiency made no mention either of the clinical state of hearing nor of the temporal bone. Nager (1921) had, however, described bony hyperplasia of the middle ear aspect of the otic capsule involving the windows of the labyrinth as part of the pathology of endemic cretinism.

Perlman and Willard's rabbit plasma vitamin A levels were 10–20 I.U. per 100 ml; the control animals had 216–340 I.U.

Only one of their sections shows nerve changes in the peripheral fibres of the basal coil, presumed to be secondary to compression of the spiral ganglion cells, though many of these ganglion cells were present. The amount of degeneration paralleled the amount of new bone formation and the degree of compression of nerve fibres in the internal auditory meatus. The hair-cells, fluid spaces of the stria vascularis all appeared normal.

Van Dyke (1942) suggested that the operation of vitamin A in this context might be via thyroid defects, and in subsequent papers showed some evidence of this, but Smith (1960) is unable to support it. Fraser (1965) found vitamin A uptake normal in two cases of Pendred's syndrome, but this offers no evidence on their state in embryonic and foetal life or in infancy.

The vitamin B group   Deficiency of the vitamin B group has from time to time been incriminated under a vague heading of perceptive deafness and presbyacusis without demonstration that it is low in the serum of the patients affected, but more serious work exists. Denny-Brown (1947) examined 3,667 returned prisoners of war who had multiple B-group deficiencies, with some neurological afflictions. Thirteen had nerve deafness among their signs. Covell (1937) found myelin degeneration of the eighth nerve in rats and chicks on various deficient diets (A, B, nicotinic acid, B_6 and vitamin C). The basal turn of the cochlea was the most affected; in nicotinic acid deficiency it was the most pronounced of all. Hair-cells were affected, and it is difficult to see how Selfridge's (1939, 1940) cases improved on treatment. Yassin and Taha (1963) studied twenty-five pellagrins without middle-ear disease and found that seven had a perceptive deafness.

Vitamin B_{12} (cobalamine) does, however, merit serious attention in this connection, for it is recognised as essential not only for normoblastic erythropoiesis but also for the maintenance of normal central nervous system function. Retinal disease due to its deficiency is also recognised. 'Tobacco amblyopia' is now considered to occur more frequently where there is already a B_{12} deficiency: cyanides of tobacco are detoxicated in the liver and converted to harmless thiocyanates by hydroxycobalamine, for which the source is B_{12}. (Lerman and Feldman, 1961; Heaton, 1962; Freeman and Heaton, 1961). The retrobulbar neuritis of pernicious anaemia can, however, appear in men or women non-pipe smokers: this appears unusual, but argues the importance of the B_{12}. Bjorkenheim (1966) has described optic atrophy in *Diphyllobothrium latum* infestation, in which only 2 per cent show a megaloblastic anaemia but 30 per cent may have neurological damage (Palva, 1962).

Like arterial disease, low serum values for B_{12} are not uncommon after middle age and are due as a rule not to dietary factors but to auto-antibodies against the gastric secretory cells.

Nigerian degenerative neurological disease

This disease of adults with advanced neurological disorder includes optic atrophy and perceptive deafness. Monekosso and Wilson (1966) suggest that a high dietary cyanide intake in a malnourished population may be a contributory factor. Comparison of thiocyanate plasma levels in such patients with those of control groups confirm that these patients had a high cyanide intake. These patients ate cassava, the principal source of dietary cyanide. Thiocyanate is the principle detoxification product. It it known that B_{12} is concerned in this metabolic aspect, and that cyanide may produce neuropathological changes in animals (Smith, 1962). Interest in the relationship has been renewed by the recognition that Leber's hereditary optic atrophy may result from an error of cyanide metabolism (Wilson, 1962).

Jamaican neuropathy

Hinchcliffe and Miall (1965) found an inexplicably high number of Jamaican subjects with unexplained sensorineural loss of hearing, in a rural community. Retrobulbar neuritis is also found in Jamaicans in hundreds of cases of poor vision. Jamaican neuropathy is a syndrome including pyramidal tract, and posterior columnar cord lesions, with sclerotic peripheral nerve lesions of a root distribution, retrobulbar neuropathy and sensorineural hearing loss. Ashcroft *et al.* (1967) report an investigation of these factors among patients in a mixed community, with no further light on the aetiology of this disease. They suggest, following Montgomery *et al.* (1964), that avitaminosis and dietary factors may be at work. The suggestion of Hill (1951, 1953) that widely consumed bush teas are the origin of the toxins responsible for veno-occlusive disease of the liver is, unfortunately, not discussed by Ashcroft *et al.* Hill *et al.* (1958) have shown that monocrotaline, one of the Senecio (ragwort) alkaloids, can produce this condition in rats. It is not clear what other dietary factors such as malnutrition are involved, but it is clear that toxic factors are not uncommonly ingested in rural populations.

References

Ashcroft, M.T., Cruikshank, E.K., Hinchcliffe, R., Jones, W.I., Miall, W.E., and Wallace, J. (1967), *W. Ind. Med. Jl. 16*, 233.
Bjorkenheim, B. (1966), *Lancet, 1*, 688.
Carroll, F.D., and Ireland, P.E. (1935), *Arch. Otolaryng. 21*, 489.
Covell, W.P. (1940), *Laryngoscope, 50*, 632.
Flesch, M. (1882), *Arch. f. Ohrenh. 18*, 65.
Fraser, G.R. (1965), *Ann. Hum. Genet. 28*, 201.
Freeman, A.C., and Heaton, J.M. (1961), *Lancet, 1*, 908.
Heaton, J.M. (1962), *Trans. Ophthal. Soc. U.K. 82*, 263.
Hill, K.R., Rhodes, K., Stafford, J.L., and Aub, R. (1953), *Brit. Med. Jl. 1*, 117.
Hill, K.R., Stephenson, C.F., and Filshie, I. (1958), *Lancet, i*, 623.
Hinchcliffe, R., and Miall, W.E. (1965), *W. Ind. Med. Jl. 14*, 241.
Lerman, S., and Feldman, A.L. (1961), *Arch. Ophthalm. 65*, 381.
Loch, W.E. (1939), *Monatschr. f. Ohrenheilk. 73*, 542.
Manasse, P. (1908), *Ver. Deutschen Otol. Ges. 17*, 185.
Mellanby, E. (1938), *J. Physiol. 94*, 380.
Monekosso, L., and Wilson, J. (1966), *Lancet, i*, 1062.
Montgomery, R.D., Cruickshank, E.K., Robertson, W.B., and McMenemey, W.H. (1964), *Brain, 87*, 425.
Moos, S., and Steinbrugge, H. (1882), *Z. Ohrenheilk. 11*, 48.
Nager, F.R. (1921), *Z. Ohrenheilk. 80*, 107.
Palva, I. (1962), *Acta Med. Scand.*, supp., 374.
Perlman, H.B. (1944), *Ann. Otol. 53*, 267.
Perlman, H.B., and Willard, J. (1941), *Ann. Otol. 50*, 349.
Selfridge, G. (1939), *Ann. Otol. 48*, 39, 419, 608.
— (1940), *Ann. Otol. 49*, 674.

Smith, A.D.M., Duckett, S., and Waters, A.H. (1963), *Nature*, Lond.
    200, 179.
Smith, J.F. (1960), *Q. J. Med. 29*, 297.
Van Dyke, J.H. (1942), *Anat. Rec. 82*, 451.
Whetnall, E. (1964), in Whetnall, E., and Fry, D.B., *The Deaf Child*,
    Heinemann, London.
Wilson, J. (1963), *Clin. Sci. 29*, 505.
Yassin, A., and Taha, M. (1963), *J. Laryng. 77*, 992.

XIII Vascular disease

The vertebral artery is the main and possibly the sole supply to the membraneous cochlea. Ischaemic lesions may be due to occlusion, whether sudden, as in embolism, or gradual, as in atheroma. Other lesions, such as syphilis, may occur; also polyarteritis nodosa and giant-celled arteritis. Too often local lesions have been looked for microscopically when the vertebral artery remained unexamined. Levine *et al.* (1949), Morris *et al.* (1962) and Bradshaw and McQuaid (1963) have pointed out that the vertebral-basilar insufficiency syndromes are not uncommon. Crowe, Guild and Polvogt (1934) found no parallel between degenerative disease in the cochlea and arteriosclerosis, but Wolff (1949) showed some. Vertebral-basilar syndromes of insufficiency may be occlusive, or partially so, or due to temporary spasm. Only four minutes' deprivation of oxygen is sufficient for permanent damage in the central nervous system. Anaemia and increased blood viscosity would also play a part where blood flow was reduced.

Polyarteritis nodosa In polyarteritis nodosa peripheral nerve lesions may be caused by lesions of the small nutrient arteries. Microscopically, the lesions consist of leucocytic infiltration in which eosinophils can be seen. Many such lesions are asymptomatic. The aetiology is a hypersensitivity. Giant-celled arteritis, in which eosinophils are rare, is a disease of the elderly and is usually painful, affecting the temporal arteries most commonly. It may cause blindness, and Cooke *et al.* (1946) report labyrinthine disturbance, including deafness. Histologically, the giant-cells and infiltration of the media by monocytes, and absence of eosinophils, make it very distinct from polyarteritis.

The vascular stria may show a variety of lesions. Von Fiendt and Saxen (1937) have shown the increasing thickness and sclerosis of the vascular walls in old age, but concluded that presbyacusis was due less to this lesion than to neuronal degeneration.

Similar lesions may be seen in diabetes mellitus, and eosinophilic deposits may be found in many conditions, listed by Gussen (1968). Friedmann was the first to find the PAS-positive material characteristic of the Jervell–Lange Nielsen lesion.

The appearance of the vascular stria in virus diseases such as congenital rubella is described with the virus diseases.

Calcium deposits in the inner ear (basophilic plaques in the stria) Rollin (1934) found similar deposits to those of Kelemen (1958) in three cases: in children of $2\frac{1}{2}$ and 6 years and a man of 59 years. These died of pulmonary tuberculosis, pneumococcal peritonitis and cerebral haemorrhage. Kelemen found a calcified stria vascularis in a twenty-five day old infant with congenital toxoplasmosis. There was a cyst as well in case 3. In case 1 certainly two turns were affected. He quotes M. B. Schmidt, who had found calcium in the walls of the choroid plexus arteries in the first year of life. Hinojosa (1958) found similar changes in the offspring of a mother suffering from pseudohypoparathyroidism. (During her pregnancy she took very large doses of vitamin D daily). He goes on to say that slight deposits of a similar nature had been found in the collection of temporal bones of 'cases of otosclerosis, Paget and toxoplasmosis'. This last refers to case 1 of Kelemen (1958).

Basophilic plaques have been found by the author in four of a series of sixty-seven infant temporal bones.

The subject may well be allied to arterial wall calcium deposition, seen in hypervitaminosis D (Hass *et al.*, 1958), accumulation of acid mucopolysaccharide (Wright, 1963) and other aetiologies (Moran and Becker, 1959).

Bleeding from the birth trauma   Voss (1926) reported the presence of blood within the scala tympani in the basal turn of the cochlea in thirty cases.

Spontaneous subarachnoid haemorrhage   Subarachnoid haemorrhage is not normally clinically associated with vestibular or auditory symptoms. Holden and Schuknecht (1968) examined twelve temporal bones from fatal cases and found blood in the internal auditory meatus in all. Blood had entered the facial canal in eight ears, as far as the geniculate ganglion in four. It was also in Rosenthal's canal in seven, the modiolar spaces in seven and the osseous spiral lamina in three. It reached the macula of the saccule in seven, but never the macula of the utricle, and was in the sheath of the vestibular nerve trunk in all.

It was present in the scala tympani, especially in the ears with the largest cochlear aqueducts.

References

Bradshaw, P., and McQuaid, P. (1963), *Q. J. Med. 32*, 279.
Cooke, W.T., Cleake, P.C.P., Govan, A.D.T., and Colbeck, J.C. (1946), *Q. J. Med. 15*, 47.
Crowe, S.J., Guild, S.R., and Polvogt, L.M. (1934), *Bull. Johns Hopkins Hosp. 54*, 315.
Friedmann, I., Fraser, G.R., and Froggatt, P. (1966), *J. Laryng. 80*, 451.
Greenfield's Neuropathology, second edition (1963), Arnold, London.
Gussen, R. (1968), *J. Laryng. 82*, 41.
Hass, G.M., Trueheart, R.E., Taylor, C.B., and Stumpe, M. (1958), *Am. J. Path. 34*, 395.
Hinojosa, R. (1958), *Ann. Otol. 67*, 964.
Holden, H.B., and Schuknecht, H.F. (1968), *J. Laryng. 82*, 321.
Kelemen, G. (1958), *Arch. Otolaryng. 68*, 547.
Levine, B., Cheskin, L.J., and Appelbaum, I.L. (1949), *Arch. Int. Med., 84*, 431.
Moran, J.J., and Becker, S.M. (1959), *Am. J. Clin. Path. 31*, 517.
Morris, A., Barton, E.K., Goldenburg, S., and Blumenthal, H.T. (1962), *Circulation, 25*, 663.
Rollin, H. (1934), *Arch. Ohr.-Nas. Kehl. 138*, 1.
Von Fiendt, H., and Saxen, A. (1937), *Acta Otolaryng.*, supp., 23.
Voss, O. (1926), *Kinderheilk, 34*, 568.
Wolff, D. (1949), *Trans. Amer. Opth. and Otol. 54*, 37.
Wright, I. (1963), *J. Clin. Path. 16*, 499.

XIV Neurological degenerative disorders

Deafness as part of the syndrome of primary neuropathy

Carcinoma Denny-Brown (1948) described the pathology of this syndrome. One of the two cases had a severe right perceptive deafness. The pathology of the cochlea and eighth nerve is not dealt with by Denny-Brown, but the general pathology is detailed as follows.

There was very severe degeneration of the dorsal columns of the spinal cord, without inflammatory reaction, and the degeneration was thus consistent with simple Wallerian degeneration of the central processes of the dorsal nerve roots, which in turn were severely degenerated. Hardly a single dorsal root cell remained in the lumbar dorsal root ganglia, again without signs of inflammation.

In a sensory nerve no intact myelin sheath remained.

Motor end plates and nerves were normal, but unexpected changes were found in muscle. (No clinical weakness had existed.) There was proliferation of sarcolemmal nuclei and increased cellularity of the connective tissue of a kind seen in chronic myositis, without the lymphorrhages of acute myositis.

Denny-Brown considered that these changes were due to a metabolic disorder related to the tumour cells, for the neuromuscular condition reproduced changes seen in pantothenic acid and vitamin E deficiency in animals.

Hodgkin's disease Buffin (1967) has reported a case of neurological disorder in a young man, including perceptive deafness and vertigo, which appeared to be part of an illness found six months later to be malignant Hodgkin's sarcoma. In considering the differential diagnosis he suggests that local deposits (or a metabolic disturbance) were unlikely and that a viral infection is more probable, the patient's immune state being disturbed many weeks before the illness declared itself, and making predisposition to infection likely. It may have occurred following, and been facilitated by continued use of, cortisone for a condition previously diagnosed as an ophthalmic perivasculitis one year earlier. Certainly, once the neurological symptoms occurred progressive deterioration was rapid. The part the viral infection played in producing malignant change in a patient with a disturbance of immunity must remain unanswered.

Though patients with Hodgkin's disease stand a 30 per cent risk of developing neurological complications, perceptive deafness does not figure very frequently. The complications are held to be due to:

cerebral local meningoencephalitis
multifocal cranial nerve palsies; third, fourth, sixth, seventh
spinal cord transverse or ascending myelitis
polyneuropathy
mononeuritis, e.g. recurrent laryngeal or brachial palsies
myalgia
myopathy, polymyositis type

No lymphoid tissue exists in the central nervous system—though deposits of malignant Hodgkin's sarcoma may occur there. Haematological and immunological effects are the likely media of such damage, e.g. by purpuric haemorrhages, platelet thromboses, anaemia. Excessive B_{12} consumption, or other nutritional effects, by the tumour would reduce available B_{12} for the specialised nerve endings, as in tobacco amblyopia, and might occur in any malignant disease. Liability to infection through altered immune mechanisms must also be considered, particularly for viruses, protozoa and fungi, which are normally of low virulence but have been described as opportunistic by Symmers (1965).

The incidence of cortical cerebellar degeneration, peripheral neuropathy and polymyositis is probably larger in Hodgkin's disease and other malignant lymphomas than in other forms of cancer, including cancer of the lung.

Hutchinson et al. (1958) point out that most neurological lesions in Hodgkin's disease resemble sub-acute combined degeneration of the cord more than any known vitamin deficiency. Their forty-five cases with neurological signs out of 229 cases of Hodgkin's disease (some 20 per cent) contained no cases of perceptive deafness, and few involving any cranial nerve.

Sarcoidosis   Gristwood (1958) reports a case of bilateral nerve deaf-ness in a patient with sarcoid, and summarizes the possible aetiology as follows:

Toxaemia affecting the hair cells.
Pressure on auditory nerve by deposits of sarcoid tissue.
Invasion of the nerve itself by the same.
Infiltration of brain-stem by perivascular collection of sarcoid tissue.

This case was improved in hearing by treatment with cortisone and anti-tuberculous drugs, though the vestibular reactions remained severely disturbed.

The rarity of eighth nerve involvement in sarcoid is shown. Facial paralysis is common—50 per cent of nervous system involve-ment, according to Colover (1948). Nerve deafness has not been reported in sarcoidosis of childhood, and in 118 cases of sarcoidosis involving the nervous system Colover found eight cases, with four cases in which the vestibular branch was involved.

Gristwood summarises twelve cases from the literature and reports a thirteenth. Only in the case he describes was the onset of deafness prior to other manifestations of disease. Histological evidence is scanty, but in the two cases (Zollenger and Mayenburg, 1941; Erickson, Odom and Stern, 1942) where there is central nervous system histology, perivascular cuffing by epithelioid cells was found in brain stem, cerebral hemispheres and cerebellum in the one, and in the pons, cerebellum and pia arachnoid of the other, in which also were plasma cells and giant cells and round cells.

Eight of the thirteen cases had facial palsy, three of them bilateral. These were mostly associated with parotid swellings, and there is no distinction between upper and lower motor nervous types of lesion, but the recovery of some is suggestive of the lower.

It is possible that altered immunity predisposed to viral infections of the eighth nerve. The seventh nerve probably has transient pres-sure problems, and need not be related aetiologically to viral infec-tion. This fits the difference in incidence of affection of the two cranial nerves.

A primary cerebellar cortical degeneration in a case of malignant lymphoma with malabsorption which did not present with diarrhoea has been described by Missen (1966), who advances the following

possibilities in the search for an explanation of neuropathies associated with malignancy and reticulo-endothelial disease:

1. Deposition of ceroid lipofuscin in intestinal mucosa leading to
   alpha-tocopherol deficiencies.
2. Toxins secreted by the abnormal tissue.
3. Utilisation of an essential metabolite by abnormal tissue.
4. Induction of auto-immune processes against central nervous
   system tissue.
5. Development of tumour might involve or facilitate introduction of infection to the body.

   (a) A potentially neurotropic virus.
   (b) 'Passenger virus' might multiply in the tumour.

6. There might be massive replacement of the lymphoreticulo-
   endothelial system, such as to impair the normal mechanism of
   immunity. 'Opportunistic infections', mentioned above, would
   be encouraged.
   See also Brain and Norris (1965).

Ageing and presbyacusis

Lipofuscin ('wear-and-tear' pigment) has long been identified by
pathologists with ageing. Ishii *et al.* (1967) have identified it in increasing quantities in older subjects in inclusions within the epithelial cells lining the endolymphatic space in the cochlea, and also in
the vestibular system. They considered it relative to lysosomal
activity. It was associated with sites of alkaline phosphatase activity,
which was not age-dependent, and other lysosomal enzymes, i.e.
β-glucuronidase, and N-acetyl-glucosaminidase. The lipofuscin
granules were not found before 6 years of age.

They were found in the apical cytoplasm of all epithelial cells
lining the endolymphatic space, sensory hair-cells, Deiter's cells,
Hensen's cells, and Claudius' cells, and the pillar cells. They were
also present in the vestibular epithelium.

Neuronal degeneration in the basal turn of the cochlea increases
with age (Bredberg, 1968).

Vascular disturbances (see chapter XIII) are also discussed, particularly with reference to haemorrhage and to basilar-artery spasm

by Hallberg (1956) and by Bradshaw and McQuaid (1963) respectively.

It may be that changes known in the retinal blood vessels increasing with age, such as micro-aneurysms, and the new capillary loops of diabetes, may also occur in the cochlea. The 'colloid bodies' of sclerosis of retinal vessels certainly resemble the eosinophilic 'globular deposits' seen in the cochlea and saccule from time to time.

Ménière's disease

Prosper Ménière described paroxysmal attacks of vertigo associated with unilateral tinnitus and deafness in 1861. Hallpike and Cairns (1938) demonstrated the existence of endolymphatic hydrops, and consequent degeneration of the sensory elements, but no satisfactory aetiology has been advanced for the disease. As Friedmann (1966) points out, similar changes may be found in for example, tuberculous meningitis.

Superficially resembling the endolymphatic hydrops of late-onset congenital syphilitic deafness, it differs in detail considerably—the syphilitic hydrops being apparently secondary to bony disease involving the otic capsule, and chronic inflammatory tissue which partially 'heals' with bony erosion.

Lindsay (1967) has described two cases in which hydrops was limited to the cochlea.

For further discussion on this interesting disease, see Dix and Hallpike (1952), Cawthorne (1956), Cawthorne and Hallpike (1957).

Friedmann, Cawthorne and Bird (1965) follow the Friedmann *et al.*'s (1963) report of finding laminated inclusions in the degenerating sensory epithelium of human utricular macula, by a description of four more cases with similar findings. They point out, however, that such inclusions may be present in patients not suffering from Ménière's disease but from eighth nerve tumour, as reported by Hilding and House (1964).

Jenkner and Vojacek (1967) found evidence of unilateral cerebrovascular damage in an investigation of a group of patients with Ménière's syndrome. Oppenheimer (1923) considered vasomotor disturbance, and sometimes atheromatosis, to be the cause of the disease. Jenkner and Vojacek examined 200 patients, forty-nine of them known to be Ménière's sufferers, who had some of the symptoms of the disease by a technique they call rheoencephalography, which records electrical resistance changes in the cerebral hemisphere in response to blood content. They found it possible to differentiate three groups, cerebral arteriosclerosis, cerebrovascular insufficiency and unilateral cerebrovascular damage. The last group was found to correspond exactly with the cases of Ménière's disease. These authors, alas, do not give any description of what precisely they mean by unilateral vascular damage.

Means, De Groot and Stanbury (1966) who point out that deafness and vertigo may also be the presenting symptoms of hypothyroidism, recommend exclusion of this by investigation of the basal metabolic rate. Poulsen (1966) claims that those with a low BMR improve on thyroxine.

References

Bradshaw, P., and McQuaid, P. (1963), *Q. J. Med. 32*, 279.
Brain, W.R., and Norris, F.H. (1965), *Brain, 88*, 465.
Bredberg, G. (1968), 'Cellular pattern and nerve supply in the human organ of Corti', *Acta Otolaryng.*, suppl., 236.
British Medical Journal, 1965, *I*, 943 (extensive bibliography).
Buffin, J.T. (1967), *J. Laryng. 81*, 1131.
Cawthorne, T.E. (1956), *J. Laryng. 70*, 695.
Cawthorne, T.E., and Hallpike, C.S., (1957), *Acta Otolaryng. 48*, 89.
Colover, J. (1948), *Brain, 71*, 451.
Denny-Brown, D. (1948), *J. Neurol. Neurosurg. Psychiatr.*, new series, *11*, 73.
Dix, M.R., and Hallpike, C.S. (1957), *Proc. Roy. Soc. Med. 45*, 241.
Friedmann, I., McLay, K., Cawthorne, T., and Bird, E.S. (1963), *J. Ultrastruct. Res. 9*, 123.
Friedmann, I., Cawthorne, T., and Bird, E.S. (1965), *J. Ultrastruct. Res. 12*, 92.
Friedmann, I. (1966), in *Systemic Pathology*, ed. Payling, Wright, and Symmers, W.StC., Longmans, London, p. 1667.
Gristwood, R.E. (1958), *J. Laryng. 72*, 479.
Hallberg, E.O. (1956), *Laryngoscope, 66*, 1237.
Hallpike, C.S., and Cairns, J. (1938), *J. Laryng. 53*, 625.
Hilding, D.A., and House, W.F. (1964), *Laryngoscope, 74*, 1135.
Hutchinson, E.C., Leonard, B.J., Maudsley, C., and Yates, P.O. (1958), *Brain, 81*, 75.

Ishii, T., Murakami, Y., Kimura, R.S., and Balogh, K., Jr. (1967), *Acta Otolaryng.* *64*, 17.
Jenkner, F.L., and Vojacek, E. (1967), *Acta Otolaryng.* *64*, 429.
Lindsay, J.R., Kohut, R.I., and Sciarra, P.A. (1967), *Ann. Otol.* *76*, 1.
Means, J.H., De Groot, L.J., and Stanbury, J.B. (1967), *The Thyroid and its diseases*, third edition, McGraw-Hill.
Missen, G.A.K. (1966), *Guy's Hosp. Rep.* *115*, 359.
Poulsen, H. (1966), in *Hormones and Connective Tissue*, ed. G. Asboe-Hansen, Munksgaard, Copenhagen.
Symmers, W.StC. (1965), *Proc. Roy. Soc. Med.* *58*, 341.

XV Infections which may lead to hearing loss

i Pathogens and defences

Pathogenic organisms have their own characteristics which determine virulence, site of attack and possible lines of spread. They also carry one or more specific antigens, and perhaps group antigens, which excite one form of response—the production of humoral antibody—from the patient. Locally, the invasion of the patient may be modified by anatomical considerations, such as intact skin, or a healthy ciliated mucosa repeatedly cleansed by flowing mucus containing lysozyme. The normal flora of the pharynx, for example, may also play an inhibitory role to the invader.

Once multiplication of a pathogen, such as *Streptococcus pyogenes*, begins in any situation, sufficient local damage occurs to call forth the inflammatory responses of the tissues. Some of these resemble the responses in sterile trauma, so that capillaries are gorged with blood products, and allow the passage of proteins and white cells to the tissue fluids surrounding the area of damage or destruction. Secretory cells may be stimulated; thus oedema, mucus and ultimately pus are present, with a highly vascular subepithelium. If the defensive mechanisms overcome the pathogens, drainage of pus must be possible: in very mild otitis media the middle ear may remain full of exudate, particularly if the otitis is aborted by antibiotics, but drainage along the eustachian tube is inadequate.

The problems of inflammation within the ear are thus those of inflammation elsewhere, with the anatomical limitations of the site.

Pathogens

Though it may be fairly true to say that acute otitis media is bacterial in aetiology, and eighth nerve and cochlear damage often viral, the distinction is not wholly true. It is proposed here to list the various groups of pathogenic organisms which may affect hearing.

PROTOZOA

Toxoplasma gondii (see chapter xix).
  Transplacental infection.

SPIROCHAETALES

Treponema pallidum (see chapter xviii).
  Transplacental infection (congenital).
  Acquired syphilis, mainly eighth nerve damage.

BACTERIA

Streptococcus pneumoniae (the pneumococcus).
  Acute infection from the pharynx.
  Secondary to meningitis.

Streptococcus pyogenes.
  Acute infection from the pharynx.

Haemophilus influenzae.
  Acute infection from the pharynx.

Neisseria meningitidis.
  Secondary to meningitis.

Pseudomonas pyocyanea, Proteus species and *Escherichia coli.*
  Presumed to be secondary invaders after acute otitis media and
    perforation of the drum.

Mycobacterium tuberculosis.
  Acute, subacute or chronic middle ear infection, possibly blood-
    borne, possibly from the nasopharynx.
  Eighth nerve damage by meningitis.

Other bacteria causing profound illness sometimes followed by
deafness are *Corynebacterium diphtheriae* and *Salmonella typhi*:
the possible pathology includes end-organ or nerve damage by
toxin, direct bacterial inflammation of the middle ear, or general
lowering of inflammatory defensive response so that invasion by
other organisms is facilitated.

VIRUSES (see chapter xvii)

Rubella virus
  Transplacental infection.
  Occasionally cochlear damage due to viraemia (post-natal).

Varicella-zoster
  Transplacental infection.
  Herpes zoster oticus.
Measles, mumps viruses and possibly *influenza* occasionally cause cochlear damage.
Para-influenza 2 and 3 and *respiratory syncytial virus* have been isolated from the middle ear in acute otitis media.

   In addition, *potential pathogens* sometimes found in the naso-pharynx which ought not to be neglected in the microbiology of the middle ear, and which would require a search by special methods:

PROTOZOA
Hartmanella species (soil amoebae).

SPIROCHAETALES
Treponema vincenti, T. microdentium, etc.

BACTERIA
Bacteroides species (gram-negative anaerobes).
Myobacterium leprae.

MYCOPLASMATA

VIRUSES

FUNGI, which are not further mentioned.
Aspergillus niger and other species.
   Secondary invaders in a chronic mastoid cavity only.
Candida albicans has been described (McLellan *et al.*, 1965) in the middle ear of a premature infant, and is frequently isolated from the pharynx.

Defence

The general defences against infection are the white cells, the histiocytes (macrophages), and the humoral antibodies. Generally speaking, a polymorphonuclear response is to be expected in bacterial infections, and lymphoid in viral infections. Bacterial otitis media is no exception.
   Antibody production is really protein synthesis by lymphoid or plasma cells, in response to specific stimulation by foreign sub-

stances. These cells share with other manufacturing cells, such as those of the pancreatic acini, a highly developed endoplasmic reticulum. This organelle appears to be the site of antibody synthesis. The cells may be distributed throughout the reticuloendothelial system, the lymph nodes, spleen, tonsils, Peyer's patches and thymus. This last has some control at the beginning of life over the development of the ability to respond to foreign protein. Lymph nodes will normally be the first active recipients of invasion via the skin; adenoids and tonsils of the mouth and nasopharynx, and Peyer's patches in the gut.

Two main types of antibody exist: cellular, where the lymphocyte carries a cell-bound site for interaction at the cell surface, and the humoral antibodies which are immunoglobulins G, A, M, D and E.

The cell-bound antibodies mediate the 'delayed hypersensitivity' response of, for example, the Mantoux test. The ability to produce these is present in the full-term human infant. Other examples are drug allergy, homograft rejection, bacterial allergy and contact hypersensitivity. Its significance as a defence mechanism is not wholly understood.

The humoral antibodies, the Gamma-globulins (see Altmeier and Smith, 1965).

A, or Gamma A or Beta$_2$ A or IgA. This is the principal immunoglobulin of the secretions of the respiratory tract, milk, colostrum, saliva, or the intestinal tract. Clearly, it is suitably located to be destined to play a useful role in defence against viral and other infections: nasal secretions in adults have been found to contain specific A long after recovery from an infection. It is a 7S or 13S protein. It is involved in histamine release.

IgG, Gamma G, an entirely 7S protein, is not normally found in secretions. It does cross the placenta, and is the only gamma-globulin to do so. It appears in nasal secretions during a primary (non-immune) infection, and in immune reactions it seems probable that the Gamma A reaction which is involved with histamine release causes a change in capillary permeability so that IgG can be released to the secretions, and there act in its specific antiviral neutralising capacity.

IgM, Gamma M is distinguished by its extremely high molecular weight. It is also the first type of antibody synthesised by the infant. It is a 19S protein.

A normal response to acute infection may begin by the production of 19S antibodies, i.e. IgM, and go on to 7S antibody. As the antigen disappears, so does the 19S protein: the 7S protein appears later in the anamnestic reaction.

Neonatal antibody formation is usually 19S, and the infant cannot synthesise 7S antibody till the third month of life (Smith, 1960).

Foetal antibodies in rubella and other congenital infections   Both types (7S and 19S) are present in the cordblood of affected newborns (Alford *et al.*, 1967) and during hysterotomy for rubella-affected pregnancy termination; 7S found in the foetus must be maternal. It can cross the placenta. 19S, if present—and it is present by the time of birth in the presence of infection—must be manufactured by the foetus. It cannot, therefore, be claimed that either immunological incompetence or tolerance accounts for the persistence of the rubella virus after birth.

The mechanism of pathogenesis of the characteristic defects of rubella is far from clear: persistence of the virus may allow damage to different systems at different times in spite of antibody. Töndury (1964) considers that embolism of rubella-infected embryonic vascular endothelium may explain some of the features most difficult to account for, such as the occasional occurrence of unilateral deafness in congenital rubella.

In the adult the antibody-producing system responds to foreign or 'not-self' antigens, but the new-borns of many species have an immature lymphoid system without antibody-producing cells. This is not because it is immunologically incompetent, but simply due to not having received antigens because of an efficient placental barrier.

Congenital syphilis and toxoplasmosis have both been shown (Silverstein, 1962) to be associated with immunological response in the foetus as early as six months' gestation.

In the absence of infection there is no gamma globulin synthesis in the foetus, which receives its IgG by transfer from maternal serum. This level starts falling one to three months after birth, later rising to adult levels. IgM is produced by the foetus two to three months after birth, and IgA after the third month. Earlier post-natal appearance of IgM and IgA thus imply exposure to antigens, and this has been used as an indication of new-borns with a high risk of infection (Alford *et al.* 1967).

The placenta   Although the placenta produces hormones, it does not produce immune bodies. The human placenta is interstitial, resulting from growth of the fertilised ovum in the uterine endometrium: this is also true of guinea-pigs. It is an invasive placenta, so that ultimately the foetal and maternal circulations are separated by a thin cellular layer, through which many substances can pass. The foetal villi are bathed in maternal blood, and the level of Gamma-G globulin in the foetal circulation is the same as or higher than the maternal level.

Circumstances affecting transmission of organisms from mother to foetus may include the level of virus-neutralising antibodies in the mother, and the number of organisms circulating during the viraemia. The transmission of protozoa clearly includes other factors, as toxoplasmosis may be transmitted from a mother no longer in the acute stage of infection.

In the guinea-pig the placenta failed to act as a barrier at any stage of pregnancy, provided that the sow had no circulating antibody. Even in the presence of such antibody it was possible to obtain some infected foetuses, when the sow had been inoculated some months previously (Wright, unpublished).

References

Alford, C.A., Schaefer, J., Blankenship, W.J., Straumfjord, J.V., and Cassady, C. (1967), *New Eng. J. Med.* 277, 438.
Altemeier, W.A., and Smith, R.T. (1965), *Ped. Clin. N. Amer.* 12, 663.
McLellan, M.S., Strong, J.P., Williams, P.M., and Baker (1965), *Arch. Otolaryng.* 82, 612.
Silverstein, A.M. (1962), *Nature*, Lond. 194, 196.
Smith, R.T. (1960), in Ciba symposium on *Cellular Aspects of Immunity*, Boston, Little, Brown.
Töndury, V.G. (1964), *Schweiz. Med. Wiss.* 20, 379.
Wright, I. (unpublished).

XVI Infections which may lead to hearing loss
ii Middle-ear and mastoid infections

Acute otitis media

Site The middle ear is continuous with the upper respiratory tract, and must be considered as much an extension of it as, for example, the maxillary antrum. It seems clear from Sadé's work (1966, 1967) that the tall, columnar, ciliated lining of the eustachian tube is continued into the middle ear, and is there replaced by a lower but still ciliated epithelium for a varying area. Mastoid air cells too have been found with a tall, columnar, secretory and ciliated lining, at least in the presence of infection (Friedmann, 1963). The processes of cleansing the cavity of any debris such as desquamated cells are therefore likely to be similar to those of the antrum, a continuous stream of moisture, likely to be mucoid, sweeping towards the opening of the eustachian tube and thence to the nasopharynx. It has long been observed that a few white cells may be seen in the middle ear, and a few macrophages. These may travel in the stream of mucus or may migrate through the epithelium. The epithelium itself is capable of taking up dyes and particulate matter.

Factors to be considered in the inflammatory response and its mobilisation are fully dealt with by Spector and Willoughby (1963) and Harris (1960). Wright (1961) has reviewed the structure and function of the respiratory tract in relation to infection, and Bang (1961) the mucociliary function as a protective mechanism. Hatch (1961) discusses the fate of particles in the respiratory tract.

The problem of pathogenic microbes obtaining access to the middle ear must therefore be bound up with dysfunction of normal tubal drainage: obstruction, such as nasopharyngitis, and lymphoid hypertrophy might play a part. Oedema and damage to the ciliary mechanism by unsuitable pH or dryness most certainly would be expected to.

Invasion This depends on the multiplication of organisms of a virulent acquired infection in the pharynx, such as *Streptococcus pyogenes*, or possibly some local encouragement to spread or a newly acquired virulence of an organism which is already 'carried' in the site, living with the normal flora. It is possible that damage to the mucosa by a virus, or by a change in the normal flora, may be encouraging factors. Obviously, extreme vitamin A deficiency would alter the character of the mucosa so as to encourage infection. Further factors often advanced are the SO_2 content of the inhaled air, and other substances of air pollution, for upper respiratory tract bacterial and some viral infections appear commoner in the winter, when air pollution is worst: the air pollution is aggravated by increased humidity and cold as well as actual increase in the products of power stations and domestic fuels.

The findings of two years' bacteriological investigation of acute otitis media and its seasonal incidence have been discussed (Wright, 1970) in relation to other upper respiratory tract infections, inclement weather and other factors: all especially pneumococcal infections increase when air pollution is high, but this must be seen in relation to cold and wet weather, which causes indoor crowding, where relative humidity may be too low for the upper respiratory mucosa.

The types of the invading organism are relevant in two ways: some are associated with particular varieties of pathogenicity, but more important is that immunity is type-specific. Some types may be more prone to invade the middle ear than others. but the important factor is probably whether the patient has yet had the opportunity to make antibody to that type.

It is interesting to see that Siirala (1957) found no evidence of inhibitory effect on *Haemophilus influenzae* in eighty-one samples of 'sterile otitis media' fluid, whereas 53 per cent of 437 samples were inhibitory to *Streptococcus pyogenes*, as Bjuggren and Tunevall (1950, 1952) have associated *H. influenzae* particularly with relapsing cases of acute otitis media. These were not all capsulated strains, which are regarded as most virulent by Turk and May (1967)—who have, however, expressed doubt on the causation of acute otitis media by even these capsulated strains in the absence of meningitis. Burns and May (1967), and Holdaway and Turk (1967), have discussed the pathogenicity of *Haemophilus influenzae* in the respiratory tract, and Dadswell (1967) its role in acute otitis media. Burns and May (1967) found agreement with the presence of H_1 antibody, detected by immunoelectrophoresis, and severity of lower respiratory tract pathology. It was found in 25 per cent of simple chronic bronchitics with mucoid sputum, in 6 and 8 per cent of healthy controls and pure asthmatics, but in 69 per cent and 88 per cent of chronic bronchitics with purulent sputum and bronchiectasis respectively. H_1 antibody has not been searched for in cases of acute otitis media. Holdaway and Turk found that only 5 per cent of respiratory tract *H. influenzae* strains were typable: they found that type a strains were associated with chronic sinusitis, types e and b with adult post-operative chest infections, and type f with bronchitis or bronchiectasis. Four out of five strains from acute otitis media and five out of five from children with pneumonia were type b, usually also associated with acute fatal epiglottitis and meningitis in young children (leading article in *The Lancet*, 1967). In another series, seven out of thirty (23 per cent) strains from acute otitis media were found to be type b, and forty-nine of 115 (42 per cent) in sinusitis (Wright, 1970). Johnstone and Lawy (1967) reported three fatal cases of adult epiglottitis, and four in children, all due to type b.

Infection All the most virulent primary bacterial invaders of the middle ear are liable to be spread by person-to-person contact in saliva, nasal secretions and droplets resulting from speech and sneezing. The survival of the organisms is related to dryness or humidity or temperatures, not so much out of doors as indoors, where people congregate and exchange flora. It has long been known that the beginning of each school term excites a minor epidemic of upper respiratory tract infections. Bacterial isolation from cases of acute otitis media would support this to some extent, particularly with the streptococcus (Wright, 1970).

Organisms *Streptococcus pyogenes, Streptococcus pneumoniae* and *Haemophilus influenzae* are regarded as the most virulent of the primary bacterial invaders of the middle ear. Types of these three pathogens isolated from this site are recorded, comparison made with bacterial isolation from other sites in the upper respiratory tract and from the external ear, and seasonal variation discussed in Wright (1970).

Investigations into the bacterial flora of acute otitis media where the specimens have been obtained by aspiration through an intact drum and the bacteriological techniques are adequate are unfortunately rare. Lahikainen (1953) surveyed the literature and reported his own series of 734 samples: 81·7 per cent grew a pure culture, 1·1 per cent a mixed culture, and 17·2 per cent were sterile.

Of the 600 monomicrobic cultures:

282 (38·2 per cent) were *Diplococcus pneumoniae* (*Streptococcus pneumoniae*).
177 (24·1 per cent) were *Streptococcus pyogenes*.
24 (3·3 per cent) were *Streptococcus viridans*.
112 (15·3 per cent) were *Haemophilus influenzae*.
13 (1·7 per cent) were *Staphylococcus pyogenes*.

All the *Streptococcus pyogenes* were group A, but none was typed. The *Diplococcus pneumoniae* were typed from 239 cultures, the most frequent being type 3 ('*Diplococcus mucosus*'), 34 per cent: other types being 1 (10 per cent), 19 (10 per cent), 6 (5·9 per cent), 23 (5 per cent), types 27, 18, 7 and 5 each between 3 and 4 per cent.

A much smaller series (total number, 33) gave a more random distribution of pneumococcal types from the middle ear: types 3 and 19 five (15 per cent) each, type 14 four, and 6, 1, 23, 27, 15, 9 and 48 less often. A larger number (101) from sinusitis showed types 6 and 13 as the commonest (13 and 11 per cent); 3 7, 9, 13, 16, 17 and 22, 5–7 per cent; and 1, 4, 10, 11, 14, 18, 19, 20, 21, 23, 26, 27, 28, 35, 37, 39 with less (1–4 per cent) (Wright, 1970).

H. influenzae was not typed, nor were serological investigations undertaken. The age range of Lahikainen's cases is not stated. Feingold *et al.* (1966) attempted a more detailed survey of ninety children, and used methods for the isolation of viruses and mycoplasmata as well as bacteria (these reported by Tilles *et al.*, 1967). They also related nasopharyngeal cultures to the organisms isolated from the ear. The findings are of interest, as only 53 per cent yielded pathogenic bacteria, and these were mainly *Diplococcus pneumoniae* and *H. influenzae*, with a higher proportion of isolations under 3 years old. They make no comment on the relative absence of *Streptococcus pyogenes*. They do, however, provide (Tilles *et al.*, 1967) information on virus and mycoplasma isolations, with serological evidence in some. Only adenovirus type 3 and Coxsackie B4 were isolated, but fourfold rises in titre were found

in other children, suggesting that viral infection was a factor at the
time.

Pathology Oedema and congestion of the mucosa, and increased
secretion, are early manifestations of inflammation. White cells are
found in the exudate, and organisms may be seen. The mucosa
shows white-cell infiltration as well as oedema, and may progress
to granulation tissue. This leads to the processes of healing, which
leave thickened fibrotic membranes. The bone may be affected
early in the suppurative process (Friedmann, 1956), and small frag-
ments of necrotic bone may be found in pus from the middle ear.
New osteoid tissue may form at the edge of the granulation tissue
as slender trabeculae, later to fill the area as dense trabecular bone
(Friedmann, 1955).

Antibiotics and myringotomy have greatly reduced the complications of acute otitis media.

Complications These include lateral sinus thrombosis, and sup-
puration, which results in pyaemia: extra-dural abscess, temporal
lobe abscess, suppurative meningitis (Jeanes, 1962) and cerebellar
abscess. Pus may track from the mastoid periosteum to the subcutaneous cervical tissues, or forwards beside the eustachian tube.

Recurrent infections

Davison (1962, 1966) considers that the child with frequent upper
respiratory infections has 'either an hereditary or an acquired immunological defect, poor nutrition, or poor environment. This latter
includes poor emotional climate.'

Discussing possible pathology, he mentions all causes of eustachian obstructions, including cleft palate, lymphoid hypertrophy,
and oedema of the eustachian tube due to infection allergy or hypothyroidism. He quotes Smull, his microbiological colleague, as
having found no correlation in size of adenoid with number of
bacterial organisms per gram of tissue. The peak incidence of 240
childhood middle-ear effusion was at 5–7 years of age, with some
male preponderance. Some 20 per cent of the patients presented
'allergic' (undefined) symptoms, 'twice the prevalence of the general
population'. Ninety (37·5 per cent) had had a prior adenoidectomy,
but Davison questions the experience of the operators and holds

recurrences of middle-ear effusion rare if done by an experienced surgeon.

Good *et al.* (1960) have pointed out that the various manifestations of antibody deficiency syndrome include neutropaenia, and Davison concludes that a white cell count of 4,000/mm^3 is thus not necessarily a ground for withholding antibiotics.

Davison discusses the possibility of hypogamma-globulinaemia.

Paavolainen (1967) estimated that in Helsinki the acute otitis media morbidity in 1961 and 1962, apart from cases seen in private practice or in the municipal hospitals, fell from 3·5 per cent of the 3 year old population to 0·2 per cent of the 15 year olds. These figures seem to be in agreement with experience in other countries.

A proportion of children, however, suffer from acute recurrent attacks, and Kiviranta (1967) has investigated 173 cases in Helsinki University ENT clinic in 1965, a year in which 6,500 cases of acute otitis were seen, giving 2·7 per cent as the proportion suffering from recurrent acute otitis during the period. These figures do not alone appear to relate to individual 'follow-ups'.

Some interesting clinical findings are revealed:

> 50 per cent of cases were aged 1 and 2 years.
> 14 per cent were younger.
> 36 per cent were 3–14 years.

Number of myringotomies:

> Ten cases had had three.
> Fifty-three cases had had ten to twenty.

The youngest was twenty-five days old at the first myringotomy, and indeed ear trouble had begun long before the ages quoted above. Kiviranta considered two pathological aspects of the cases: size and distribution of the lymphatic tissue round the eustachian tube and the adenoids and tonsils, and also the distribution of plasma proteins, which he investigated in detail. No figures existing for normal infants and children in Finland, Oberman *et al.*'s (1956) are referred to for comparison.

Kiviranta could find no actual significant deviation except in the gamma-globulin fraction; he compared the values obtained in 200 cases of tonsillitis, sinusitis, pseudo-croup, adhesive otitis, etc.,

from his own clinic with Oberman *et al.*'s figures (1956) and found
equal or somewhat higher figures. The recurrent otitis patients,
however, in nearly all age groups had significantly lower gamma-
globulin levels, amounting on average to not more than two-thirds
of the 'normal values' of Oberman.

The normal increase of gamma-globulin levels with age did not
appear to take place in these groups, and Kiviranta suggests a form
of immunological paralysis secondary to the strain of recurrent infections in 1–2 year olds, manifesting itself as a standstill in the
normal continuing elevation of the gamma-globulin level.

Nevertheless, sixty-two patients received gamma-globulin after
myringotomy. The basis of selection is not wholly clear, but was
probably recurrent acute otitis media, at one week to one month
after myringotomy, between the ages of 6 months to 2 years, which
did not respond to antibiotic treatment.

Clinically the results appeared worthwhile, though there were
some relapses at 3–6 months.

Viral infection of the middle ear

Respiratory syncytial virus (RSV)   This virus defied identification
for many years because it is destroyed by refrigeration and is thus
best isolated by direct inoculation. For details of inoculation and
types of cells, see Berglund *et al.* (1966).

Berglund *et al.* (1967) investigated groups of children in the
autumn of 1966, when RSV was known to be prevalent in the city
of Turku. They selected thirty-three children with acute respiratory
tract infection and collection of fluid in one or both ears. Their
ages ranged from three months to four years. All were subjected to
venepuncture to provide paired specimens of serum which were
later investigated not only for evidence of rising antibody against
RSV but also for complement-fixing antibody against other viruses,
and 'Eaton's agent' (*Mycoplasma pneumoniae*).

Pharyngeal swabs were also obtained, and cell cultures inoculated
at the same time as the inoculation with fluid from the middle ear.
Of those eighteen children who had RSV in the pharynx, seven
had a positive aspirate for one or both ears. Of the thirty-four
aspirates of two groups, eleven (39 per cent) were positive for RSV.
This is a lower percentage than was isolated during the spring

study (Berglund *et al.*, 1966), which amounted to 76 per cent (confined to a study of children up to 12 months in both groups, the discrepancy is greater, 87 per cent in the spring and 25 per cent in the autumn).

Of those fifteen children with negative throat swabs, none yielded RSV or other virus from the middle-ear aspirate.

Berglund *et al.* (1967) consider that the virus may achieve access to the middle ear in mucus, and comments on the similarity of the low cuboidal normal middle-ear lining cell to that of the alveolar cells. Shedden and Emery (1965) have demonstrated RSV in bronchial, bronchiolar and alveolar epithelium of infants dying of giant-cell bronchitis, a severe respiratory tract infection. Berglund *et al.* (1967) consider the virus capable of reproducing in the cells of the ostium of the eustachian tube and in the cavum tympani.

Abundant mucus production is a feature of RSV infections in other situations, hence this virus should be considered under 'glue ear', *q.v.*

Berglund *et al.* (1967) noted that one child who was in their spring *and* autumn series suffering from RSV virus had virus isolation in the spring from the pharynx, when he had bronchopneumonia and bilateral reddened, bulging ear-drums, and again in the autumn, when he was hospitalised with cough, sinusitis, dyspnoea and high fever. The ear-drums were thickened at this time, rigid and pale, and fluid was aspirated but proved negative for virus and for bacteria. Seven days later *Haemophilus influenzae* was isolated from the left ear, and RSV had disappeared from the pharynx. The CF titre against RSV had risen from 1/4 to 1/64 during the second illness, and it was therefore considered that this was a second infection.

It seems clear that references to multi-nucleated giant cells in the ear must give rise to suspicion of undiagnosed RSV infection. As in the lungs, their presence has been attributed to other causes. The somewhat mysterious references to 'foreign-body otitis' must be re-examined in this light.

Shedden and Emery (1965) have shown that in the bronchioles there is little inflammatory reaction in the deeper tissues, but bizarre epithelial appearances including very large syncytial masses. Cells very suggestive of RSV infection are found in the middle ear of young children from time to time (Wright, unpublished).

Co-existence of viral and bacterial infection

This is no longer merely speculative. Grönroos *et al.* (1968) have isolated respiratory syncytial virus (RSV) and *Streptococcus pneumoniae* type XIV from the middle ear exudates of five children out of eleven with acute otitis media. This was during an RSV epidemic in a nursery, in which thirteen children were studied. The children were initially not on antibiotics, except two cases, and bacterial isolation was possible, as it had not been in Berglund *et al.*'s study (1967). RSV and other pathogens were isolated from the pharynx. Antibody titres to the relevant potential pathogens were estimated.

RS virus was isolated from the threat of every infant within the first two days of the disease, but only in three cases one week later. One case relapsed, and the virus was found in the throat on the seventeenth day. The virus was isolated from the middle ear in six children, one of whom had no accompanying bacterial agent. One had *Streptococcus viridans*.

Three children had both RSV and the pneumococcus present in the middle ear: two others had, so to speak, a virus on one side and a coccus on the other. One child had unilateral pneumococcus only: it had, of course, RSV in the throat.

Increase of antibodies in the serum to RSV in the throat was detected in all but the youngest (aged one month). Significant rises in titre were not found in children under three months old in a previous study (Berglund *et al.*, 1965) until three to four weeks of illness. Pneumococcal antibodies were not detected, or rose very little in the youngest children. This is in accordance with Tunevall's findings (1953).

Adenovirus type 2 was present in the throat of two children, and type 5 in one; significant rises in titre were found in those children. These three also had *S. pneumoniae* in the throat but no significant anti-pneumococcal titres.

Mycoplasmata and the middle ear

This group of organisms is represented in the oropharynx by (Taylor-Robinson and Purcell, 1966):

M. salivarium.
M. orale types 1 and 2

M. pneumoniae.
M. hominis type 1.
T strain (Shepard, 1954, 1956).

Of the first three, there is no evidence of causation of disease
(Kleineberger–Nobel, 1962). *M. pneumoniae* (Eaton's agent) is
responsible for 'primary atypical pneumonia' (Chanock *et al.*, 1963;
Marmion and Hers, 1963; Hayflick and Chanock, 1965; Eaton,
1965). It also has a possible role in mucocutaneous syndromes, including Stevens–Johnson syndrome (Ludlam *et al.*, 1964), and
Behcet's syndrome.

   M. hominis is found in the oropharynx of 5 per cent of normal
adults as well as in the genito-urinary tract, where its role is not
quite dissociated from non-specific urethritis, and non-gonococcal
salpingitis. T strain (Shepard, 1954, 1956) is similarly of doubtful
aetiological significance.

   Chanock and Purcell (1967) produced an exudative pharyngitis
with fourfold increase in antibody titre, with nasal instillation of
cultures of *M. hominis* type 1 into healthy male volunteers.
Some of the volunteers developed a cervical lymphadenopathy.
It must be concluded that *M. hominis* type 1 is capable of
pathogenicity in the nasopharynx, and, as those volunteers with
no pre-inoculation antibody were more prone to symptoms and to
signs of disease than those with such antibody, that such antibody
is protective.

   A pathogen or resident of the pharynx may be considered a
potential agent for middle-ear infections. No such evidence has been
reported for *M. hominis* type 1, but *M. pneumoniae* has been
isolated from cases of acute otitis media in children (Sobeslavsky
et al., 1965) and in volunteers (Rifkind *et al.*, 1962). Sobeslavsky
et al. reported three cases in children of 5, 8 and 15 years of age.
All had a mild upper respiratory tract infection, and otitis media
developed after several days. The ear-drum of the youngest child
was mildly oedematous, and covered with minute blebs filled with
a serous liquid. *M. pneumoniae* was isolated from the ear and nasopharynx of the 15 year old after eight to ten days' incubation, and
on the fourteenth day from the nasopharynx of the 5 year old; but
not from either swab of the third patient, who had no fluid in the
middle ear when paracentesis was performed.

Cold agglutinin titres were less than 1/4 in all three cases. Paired sera from the three patients showed rises in antibody, twofold (5 years), fourfold (8 years old) and sixteenfold (15 years). Commenting on the similarity of the signs in these cases and Chanock, Rifkind et al.'s human volunteers, from whose middle ears no M. pneumoniae was isolated, Sobeslavsky suggests that difference in technique may have been responsible. He did not take swabs until after paracentesis.

Rifkind and Chanock et al. (1962) used male volunteers of 21–36 years of age. Twenty-seven had no demonstrable pre-inoculation antibody and twenty-five with titres of 1/4–1/20. In the first group there were three cases of primary atypical pneumonia, one of whom also developed myringitis, and eleven further myringitis cases, with six other upper respiratory illness. Among those with pre-inoculation antibody there were no cases of pneumonia, but six of febrile respiratory illness and one myringitis. There was a fourfold rise in antibody titre in all the first group, and in seventeen of the twenty-five who had previous antibody.

Describing the myringitis, Rifkind et al. found it was usually bilateral, with throbbing pain, after an incubation period of six to nine days. The drum might be mildly infected or severely inflamed with oedema. Five of the thirteen patients developed haemorrhagic areas. Two of them proceeded to serum-filled blebs, which later also filled with blood. There was no bulging of the drum, no fluid behind it, and no spontaneous rupture. The duration of the otitis varied from three to thirteen days—four patients had a white cell count of 10–12,000 mm^3.

Dawes' (1953) description of bullous myringosa haemorrhagica, which he considered viral in origin, probably includes this type.

Bacteroides

This is an anaerobic group of gram-negative bacilli, and representatives of it are oral and pharyngeal inhabitants, incriminated as pathogens in septic oral conditions, particularly in the presence of certain other organisms such as Treponema vincenti and T. microdentium, anaerobic streptococci and diphtheroids (Socransky, MacDonald, Gibbons and co-workers, Harvard Dental School). They are also noted as being isolated in pus or in blood cultures in post-operative septicaemias (McHenry et al., 1961), and it is likely that their requirements of prolonged anaerobic culture have concealed their presence in many other cases of infection. That is to say, it is likely that only a proportion of the cases of pyrexial illness due to these organisms have been bacteraemias, because only blood cultures are usually kept in suitable conditions for a period of three weeks, and other sites would have yielded false negative results.

Himalstein (1967) has reported an osteomyelitis of the maxilla due to *Bacteroides fundibuliformis*. It had the characteristic of foul-smelling pus usually ascribed to bacteroides infections.

No report has appeared of middle-ear infections, but no adequate techniques are likely to be in routine use for isolation of these organisms. The fact that mouth and nasopharynx are the habitat suggest that invasion of the eustachian tube is possible.

Tuberculous infection of the middle ear and mastoid

This is an uncommon chronic or sub-acute disease most likely to be diagnosed by routine histology of bone chips and mastoid curettings. The age range is wide (Jeanes and Friedmann, 1960). At the Institute of Laryngology and Otology, nine tuberculous cases were diagnosed in 1953–59 in 1,490 specimens of mastoid bone chips. The generally low rate of bacteriological confirmation is probably explained by lack of material for such examination. Where a surgeon considers this as a possible diagnosis, *Mycobacterium tuberculosis* may be seen on a direct film made from the milky white fluid in the middle ear, and confirmed by culture on Loewenstein–Jensen slopes, and inoculation of a guinea-pig. Two cases were diagnosed at the Institute of Laryngology and Otology in 1962–4 (Wright, 1970).

The route of spread may be haematogenous: some of Jeanes and Friedmann's cases had pulmonary lesions. But in view of the probably not uncommon tuberculous primary lesion of the adenoids it seems likely that spread along lymphatics and possibly the lumen of the eustachian tube must be considered.

Fields (1967) has recorded an unusual and possibly unique case of bilateral tuberculous mastoiditis and cold Bezold's abscess in an infant. He regards these as primary tuberculous lesions, but does not exclude the nasopharynx as the primary site.

Leprosy (Hansen's disease)

Hansen's disease is not apparently associated in any form of disease of the middle or inner ear (Cochrane and Davey). There are instances, however, of *Mycobacterium leprae* being found in auditory schwannomata (Lumsden, 1964).

It is possible that *M. leprae* does not affect the middle ear, the cochlea or the eighth nerve; it is also likely that the possibility of its true aetiology might be overlooked in a patient so severely handicapped as a case of destructive lepromatous leprosy. The central nervous system is remarkably free from lepromatous granulomata. The seventh cranial nerve is very often affected by such a lesion.

Until recently no experimental animal has been available for showing the pathology of the disseminated disease, nor has the mycobacterium been cultivable. Only in 1960 was the production of any animal lesion by *M. leprae* reported (Shepard, 1960) after inoculation into the foot pads of mice and other rodents. The infection remains small and multiplication is scanty. The number may actually decline after eight months and again after a second peak at thirteen months, so that the proportion of non-viable forms may increase.

In patients the disease varies, possibly with size of dose, and with immune response. In mice the important factor is in the immune response, and Rees (1965, 1966) has shown that thymectomy followed by total body irradiation increases the ability of injected *M. leprae* to multiply in the foot pad. Further, lesions developed elsewhere in the nose and in the fore paws. Nodular lesions appeared and these seemed to represent more closely human disease. External ears, foot pads and cutaneous nerves were all involved, in mice which had been subjected to thymectomy and 900r. Further, viable bacilli were seen at thirteen months, in the sole-plate nuclei of motor nerves and in the neighbouring Schwann cells. Another lesion reported by Rees *et al.* (1967) is a very heavily infected mucoperichondrium in the nose of an animal infected in the hind foot pad fourteen months previously. Some of the globi had ruptured, and bacilli were leaving these on the surface of the mucosa and becoming embedded in mucus.

'Glue ear'

Exudative otitis media is a clinical entity including serous and catarrhal (mucoid) non-suppurative effusion in the middle ear.

Clinically, it presents as deafness due to fluid, which may be very viscous, hence 'glue ear'. In some untreated cases the exudate will organise and may cause deafness due to chronic adhesive otitis. It is commoner in children than in adults, and otologists claim that its prevalence is increasing. The first description of this disease is usually ascribed to Politzer (1862). James Hinton illustrated the characteristic bluish appearance of the drum, sometimes with fluid level, in his *Atlas of the Membrana Tympani* (1874). Jonathan Wathen, an eighteenth century surgeon of Devonshire Square, London, suspected that a patient 'somewhat deaf from cold, and the outer ear found clear from hardened wax' might be deaf because of mucus far up the eustachian tube. 'When this disorder is but slight and recent, nature seems to relieve herself; but when more confirmed, her efforts are ineffective for its removal.' When one of his deaf patients, a young man of 37, died of smallpox in Cold-bath Fields Hospital in August 1747, Wathen took the opportunity to confirm his suspicion of the cause of his patient's deafness. He described his findings to the Royal Society in 1755: both eustachian tubes had been 'stuffed quite full of congested mucus'. Wathen referred to Haller's description of the lining of the eustachian tube as 'full of criptae and mucous cells, continued from and like the membrane of the nares', and also to 'Moganni [*sic*] and others tell us that they constantly find the cavity of the tympanum in infants always much clogged with mucus'.

There are many theories of causation. Effusion, possibly following a 'cold', in the presence of obstruction is generally agreed, but allergy, abnormal immune responses, low altitude and high humidity, hypersecretion, the presence of secretory columnar epithelium within the middle ear, dental malocclusion, and even the presence of penicillin deposited during systemic administration, have all been considered to play a part. Viral aetiology has been proposed, also that the virulence of the pyogenic bacteria causing suppurative otitis media may be diminishing. All potential factors are discussed by Friedmann (1963), Senturia (1963) and Grahne (1964). Friedmann (1955) has shown that in the guinea-pig tall secretory columnar epithelium appears in response to infection. He considers that much of the fluid may come from these cells in cases of human middle-ear effusions.

Although myringotomy and aspiration has been an accepted

method of treatment for many years, investigation of the fluid thus obtained has often been confined to the chemical nature of its consistency, identification of its proteins and hexosamines, and the relation of its viscosity to the degree of hearing loss. Although Senturia *et al.* (1958) have understandably included 'secretory' otitis media in their consideration of the whole field of tubotympanitis, and Harrison (1967, 1969) names it *exudative otitis media*, the idea persists that there must be some special characteristic of the fluid or the local histopathology to account for the condition. Rarely cultured, the fluid has usually been described as yielding no significant bacterial growth, and such viral studies as have been undertaken have been uninformative. Cytology of the fluid obtained by aspiration from these ears has shown polymorphonuclear leucocytes, macrophages, lymphocytes and plasma cells. Yeast cells and bacteria were also seen in some. Previous descriptions have too often been concerned mainly with the presence of eosinophils (Wright and Kapadia, 1969).

Chronic otitis media

Chronic ear infections are characterised by perforation of the drum, so that a flora less related to that of the pharynx may be expected. The gram-negative bacilli appear to predominate; skin flora and fungi may frequently be present. The mucosal lining of the chronic ear is thick and fibrotic. There may be infiltration by round cells, i.e. lymphocytes and plasma cells. Ciliated columnar epithelium may be found extensively, and the secretion helps to maintain the discharge and probably supplies a medium for the encouragement of microbial growth.

Granulation tissue may protrude as an 'aural polyp'; a granuloma containing cholesterol clefts may also develop, with foreign body giant cells.

The bone of the middle ear and mastoid shows evidence of absorption and new formation. Friedmann (1956, 1957) has pointed out that the altered microscopical pattern makes a distinction between the sclerotic bone with irregular pattern of cement lines and the normal pattern of lamellar bone with regular Haversian systems.

The cholesteatoma is an epidermoid cyst in any part of the middle ear, and gradually expands internally, by desquamation, even eroding bone. The very presence of squamous epithelium within the middle ear and mastoid is abnormal, and mainly two theories account for it: one is metaplasia, secondary to chronic infection, and the other is migration of squamous epithelium through the perforation of the drum. The external auditory meatus epithelium is known to migrate physiologically, peripherally from the centre of the drum and thence to the outer ear (Alberti, 1964). Simmons (1961) followed deposited particles acting as markers near a perforation in two patients; in one, migration appeared to occur into the middle ear. Alberti (1964) refers to the work of a colleague on migration near perforations into the middle ear, but it appears to have remained unpublished.

Palva *et al.* (1968) reviewed forty-five middle ear biopsies in cases of chronic ear disease. They concluded that squamous 'resting' epithelium would form keratin: on granulation tissue it performed a covering function. Abramson (1969) has shown collagenase to be present in cholesteatomata.

References

Abramson, M. (1969), *Ann. Otol. 78,* 112.
Alberti, P.W.R.M. (1964), *J. Laryng. 78,* 808.
Bang, F.B. (1961), *Bact. Rev. 25,* 228.
Berglund, B., Vihma, L., and Wickström, J. (1965), *Am. J. Epidem. 81,* 271.
Berglund, B., Salmivalli, A., and Grönroos, J.A. (1967), *Acta Otolaryngol. 63,* 445.
Berglund, B., Salmivalli, A., and Toivanen, P. (1966), *Acta Otolaryngol. 61,* 475.
Bjuggren, G., and Tunevall, G. (1950), *Acta Otolaryng. 38,* 130.
— (1952), *Acta Otolaryng. 42,* 311.
Burns, M.W., and May, J.R. (1967), *Lancet, 1,* 354.
Chanock, R.M., Mufson, M.A., Somerson, N.L., and Couch, R.B. (1963), *Amer. Rev. Resp. Dis. 88,* supp., 218.
Chanock, R.M., and Purcell, R.H. (1967), *Med. Clin. N. Amer. 51,* 791.
Dadswell, J.V. (1967), *Lancet, 1,* 243 (and letter 442).
Davison, F.W. (1966), *Ann. otol. 75,* 735.
— (1962), *Ped. Clin. N. Amer. 9,* 4.
Dawes, J.D.K. (1953), *J. Laryngol. 67,* 313.

Eaton, M.D. (1965), *Ann. Rev. Microbiol. 19*, 379.
Feingold, M., Klein, J.O., Haslam, G.E., Tilles, J.G., Finland, M., and
   Gellis, S.S. (1966), *Am. J. Dis. Child. 111*, 361.
Fields, J.A. (1967), *Laryngoscope, 77*, 489.
Friedmann, I. (1955), *J. Laryng. 68*, 27, 588.
— (1956), *J. Clin. Path. 9*, 229.
— (1957), *J. Laryng. 71*, 313.
— (1963), *Proc. Roy. Soc. Med. 56*, 695.
Good, R.A., Zak, S.J., Condie, R.M., and Bridges, R.A. (1960), *Ped.
   Clin. N. Amer. 7*, 2.
Grahne, B. (1964), *Acta otolaryng. 58*, 1.
Grönroos, J.A., Vihma, L., Salmivalli, A., and Berglund, B. (1968),
   Acta Otolaryn. 65, 505.
Haller, quoted by Wathen (1755).
Harris, H. (1960), *Bact. Rev. 24*, 3.
Harrison, K. (1967), *Practitioner, 199*, 744.
— (1969), *Proc. Roy. Soc. Med. 62*, 456.
Hatch, T. (1961), *Bact. Rev. 25*, 237.
Hayflick, L., and Chanock, R.M. (1965), *Bact. Rev. 29*, 185.
Himalstein, M.R. (1967), *Laryngoscope, 77*, 559.
Hinton, James (1874), *Atlas of the Membrana Tympani.*
Holdaway, M.D., and Turk, D.C. (1967), *Lancet, 1*, 358.
Jeanes, A.L. (1962), *J. Laryng. 76*, 338.
Jeanes, A.L., and Friedmann, I. (1960), *Tubercle* (Lond.), *41*, 109.
Johnstone, J.M., and Lawy, H.S. (1967), *Lancet, 2*, 134.
Kiviranta, U.K. (1967), *J. Laryng. 81*, 1253.
Kleineberger-Nobel, E. (1962), *The Pleuropneumonia-like Organisms.*
Lahikainen, E.H. (1953), *Acta Otolaryng.*, supp., 107.
Leading article, *The Lancet* (1967), *1*, 369.
Ludlam, G.B., Bridges, J.B., and Benn, E.C. (1964), *Lancet, i*, 958.
Lumsden, C.E. (1964), in *Leprosy in Theory and Practice*, second edition,
   ed. R. G. Cochrane and T. F. Davey, Wright, Bristol.
Marmion, B.P., and Hers, I.F.P. (1963), *Amer. Rev. Resp. Dis. 88*, 198.
McHenry, M.D., Wellman, W.E., and Martin, W.J. (1961), *Arch. Int.
   Med. 107*, 572.
Morganni (*sic*) [Morgagni], quoted by Wathen (1755).
Oberman, J.W., Gregory, K.O., Burke, F.G., Ross, S., and Rice, E.C.
   (1956), *New Eng. J. Med. 255*, 743.
Paavolainen, M. (1967), *Acta Otolaryng.*, supp. 227, 360.
Palva, T., Palva, A., and Dammert, K. (1968), *Acta Otolaryng. 87*, 21.
Politzer, A. (1862), *Wien. Med. Wschr. 12*, 197.
Rees, R.J.W. (1965), *Internat. J. Leprosy, 33*, 646.

Rees, R.J.W. (1966), *Nature*, London, *211*, 657.
Rees, R.J.W., Waters, M.F.R., Weddell, A.C.M., and Palmer, E. (1967), *Nature*, London, *215*, 599.
Rifkind, D., Chanock, R.M., Kravetz, H.M., Johnson, K.M., and Knight, V. (1962), *Amer. Rev. Resp. Dis. 85*, 479.
Sade, J. (1966), *Arch. Otolaryng. 84*, 137, 297.
— (1967), *Arch. Otolaryng. 86*, 128.
Senturia, B.H., Gessert, C.F., Carr, C.D., and Baumann, E.S. (1958), *Ann. Otol. 67*, 440.
— (1963), *Proc. Roy. Soc. Med. 56*, 687.
Shedden, W.I.H., and Emery, J.L. (1965), *J. Path. Bact, 89*, 343.
Shepard, C.C. (1960), *J. Exp. Med. 112*, 445.
Shepard, M.C. (1954), *Am. J. Syph. 38*, 113.
— (1956), *J. Bact. 71*, 362.
Siirala, U. (1957), *Pract. Otorhinolaryng. 19*, 159.
Simmons, F.B. (1961), *Arch. Otolaryng. 74*, 435.
Smull, C. (unpublished), Geisinger Medical Center, Danville, Pa.
Sobeslavsky, O., Syrucek, L., Bruckova, M., and Abrahamovitz, M. (1965), *Pediatrics* (Springfield, Ill.), *35*, 652.
Socransky, S.S., Gibbons, R.J., Dale, A.C., Bortnick, L., Rosenthal, E., and Macdonald, J.B. (1963), *Arch. Oral. Biol. 8*, 273; also previous and subsequent papers in that journal.
Spector, W.G., and Willoughby, D.A. (1963), *Bact. Rev. 27*, 117.
Taylor-Robinson, D., and Purcell, R.H. (1966), *Proc. Roy. Soc. Med. 59*, 1112.
Tilles, J.G., Klein, J.O., Jao, R.L., Haslem, J.E., Feingold, M., Gellis, S.S., and Finland, M. (1967), *New Eng. J. Med. 277*, 613.
Tunevall, G. (1953), *Scand. J. Clin. Lab. Invest. 5*, 1.
Turk, C., and May, J.R. (1967), *Haemophilus Influenzae: Its Clinical Importance*, English Universities Press, London.
Wathen, J. (1756), *Phil. Trans. 49*, 213.
Wright, G.W. (1961), *Bact. Rev. 25*, 219.
Wright, I., and Kapadia, R. (1969), *J. Laryng. 83*, 367.
Wright, I. (1970), *J. Laryng. 84*, 283.

XVII Infections which may lead to hearing loss
iii The cochlea and the eighth nerve

The organ of Corti is susceptible to inflammation affecting the membranous cochlea, and it is convenient to consider those infections which affect it possibly directly, possibly via the stria vascularis, together with less direct cochlear damage associated with neighbouring lesions, such as labyrinthitis secondary to chronic middle ear disease, and the causation of endolymphatic hydrops in, for example, tuberculous meningitis.

Suppurative labyrinthitis

This is said to occur rarely in acute otitis media, except where the otitis media has been associated with myringitis bullosa haemorrhagica (Dawes, 1951, 1953, 1963). It can occur if the stapes has been removed or damaged, or if direct extension has taken place, even in an apparently healed middle ear cleft through a fistula left by extrusion of a cholesteatoma.

In a survey of sixty-seven routine post-mortems on infants and young children the author found evidence of one destructive cochleitis associated with acute otitis media, and several minor evidences such as excess protein in the cochlear canals, fibrin threads and some hair-cell damage in other cases of acute otitis media.

Suppurative labyrinthitis may also occur in extension of meningomyelitis.

In chronic otitis media, cholesteatomatous erosion is the commonest cause, more commonly affecting the semi-circular canals than the cochlea; the membranous labyrinth resisting destruction and becoming thickened. If an exacerbation of the middle ear infection should occur the labyrinth may suffer only a sero-fibrinous exudation, and the disease, if cured, leaves functional recovery possible. If not, then suppurative labyrinthitis occurs: occasionally a whole cochlea has sequestrated.

Endolymphatic hydrops

Endolymphatic hydrops due to obstruction of the ductus and saccus endolymphaticus by fibrosis may follow meningitis of any sort; the suppurative diseases of the meninges such as pneumococcal and meningococcal meningitis may produce this lesion. Tuberculous meningitis may also obstruct the endolymphatic flow, and possibly this mechanism is operative in hydrops of other aetiology such as syphilis (see chapter xviii). In all these diseases the possibility of cranial nerve damage is also present.

Cochleitis and neuronitis due to these causes are rarer today than formerly in Britain, and it is recognised that the viruses play a very important part, both in causing disease in the adult or child patient and in affecting the cochlea of the foetus when the mother suffers from an otopathic virus infection.

The virus as a cause of deafness

The possible role of non-bacterial pathogens in acute otitis media has been considered; it is certainly as great in cochleitis. The viruses are insusceptible to antibiotics or chemotherapy, and are associated with respiratory disease of children.

Chanock and Parrott (1965) assess bacteria as unimportant primary pathogens in the lower respiratory tract in infancy and childhood compared with the viruses. The place of non-bacterial pathogens in the upper respiratory tract has also been assessed as important by Stuart–Harris (1963). The five known groups of viruses attacking the respiratory tract are all RNA viruses, except the adenoviruses.

Adenoviruses (size 65–85 millimicrons) were recovered by Rowe *et al.* (1953) from tonsils and adenoids and by Hilleman and Werner (1954) from throats of soldiers ill with acute respiratory disease.

Parainfluenza (myxoviruses; 80–200 millimicrons) isolated from laryngo-tracheo-bronchitis, croup and pneumonia (Kuroya, 1953).

Influenza A and B (myxoviruses). These attack the ciliated mucosa of the air passages 'anywhere from the nose to the alveolus'. There is also a true viral lesion, both in experimental animals and in man, of the alveolar cells (Hers *et al.*, 1958). Secondary bacterial invasion is of course common at all sites.

Respiratory syncytial virus (Morris, 1956). Possibly the chief

cause of bronchitis, and bronchopneumonia of young infants
(Chanock *et al.*, 1962).

Picornaviruses (17–34 millimicrons), which include enteroviruses
and rhinoviruses.

Rhinoviruses (Tyrell and Parsons, 1960) occur in the nose and
pharynx.

Coxsackie and ECHO viruses can of course produce polio-like
illness, but also respiratory illness (Price, 1956), though normally
classed as enteroviruses.

Although it is apparent that the viruses may attack what are
primarily ciliated mucosae, it is clear that they are not deterred from
other zones, for example the influenza virus and the alveolar
lesion. Some viruses, any or all of these groups, have been found in
aetiological relationship to disease of the middle ear, as has already
been seen in the *Mycoplasma pneumoniae* (Eaton's agent) (Rifkind
et al., 1962). Pathogenesis might be primarily viral, or the virus
might prepare the ground for bacterial invasion and non-resistance.
Virus isolation from disease of the middle ear is not unknown.
Parainfluenza 3 and 2 viruses have been reported by Tóth *et al.*
(1965) as causative of respiratory infections accompanied by otitis
media in 42 and 11 per cent of cases respectively. Coxsackie B4 has
been isolated from otitis media (Tilles *et al.*, 1967), and an adenovirus. Respiratory syncytial virus appears able to cause otitis media
alone or with other pathogens (see chapter xvi).

Certain viruses are, however, known to attack the inner ear by
causing labyrinthitis or neuronitis, and nerve damage may appear
during allergic encephalitis following a viral infection. Dawes
(1963) lists seven groups of viruses capable of producing central
nervous system lesions, and it is reasonable to expect that eighth
nerve damage will occur in such cases from time to time:

Pox viruses
    Smallpox (variola)
    Vaccinia
    Varicella-zoster

Myxoviruses
    Mumps
    Influenza
    Adenovirus

Parainfluenza
Common cold (now grouped separately as rhinoviruses)
Respiratory syncytial virus

Enteroviruses
Polio virus
Coxsackie
ECHO

Exanthems
Measles
Rubella
Herpes simplex
Lymphocytic choriomeningitis

Rabies

Arbor
Tick, louse or mite-borne encephalitides

Hepatitis viruses

The perceptive deafness, tinnitus, vertigo, and cranial nerve palsies, may be found in encephalitis of measles, mumps, rubella and scarlet fever (Miller *et al.*, 1956, 1957), post-vaccinial, allergic and drug encephalitides. Deafness may be caused by mumps, herpes zoster or rubella before birth.

The most important of all are the congenital rubella infections. Less common are the eighth nerve damage of measles, mumps, and herpes zoster.

Epidemic labyrinthitis

Epidemic vertigo was described by Falconer (1852) and more recently by Newell Price (1956), Currie (1961), extensively analysed by Pedersen (1959) and discussed in a leading article in *The Lancet* (1952). It is usually attributed to a virus disease on the sole ground of occurrence during a known virus epidemic, and this obscurity will remain if clinicians are unable to submit relevant specimens to investigating laboratories. A negative but important contribution to the histopathology has been made by Marshall (1955), whose patient, dying eight weeks later of coronary thrombosis, was found to have a normal labyrinth.

James (1964) described six clinical cases of vertigo, in two cases accompanied by vomiting, but not involving deafness, during July–December 1963 in South Africa, when the following virus diseases were prevalent:

1. 'A form of influenza which has not been officially described, classified or even recognised by the public health authorities', but which he considered as severe as that of Asian influenza several years previously.
2. Rubella 'rampant to a degree probably unique in South African epidemiology'.
3. Mumps.
4. Chickenpox.
5. Measles.
6. Infectious hepatitis.

Sataloff and Vasallo (1968), impressed by temporary sensorineural loss, recruitment and diplacusis in several patients suffering from a cold in the head, suggest that a viral cochleitis may well occur. Viral studies were only attempted three weeks after the patients' first visit, in two of their five cases, and were negative.

Beal *et al.* (1967) described the histopathology of a case of deafness apparently following a 'cold': it corresponded histologically with previously documented cases of maternal rubella. They suggest that the virus reaches the inner ear during the viraemia, first affecting the stria vascularis.

Lindsay (1967) describes deafness associated with adult cases of respiratory infection as milder than those of maternal rubella, with measles or with other viruses, and confined to the contents of the cochlear canal: the findings (Beal *et al.*) were consistent with those in which a viral origin was definite. They also seemed to correspond with some of Schuknecht's (1962) cases.

Infectious mononucleosis

Gregg and Shaeffer (1964) reported a case of sudden onset of inner-ear type of deafness and labyrinthine disturbance during the active stage of infectious mononucleosis in a man of 17 years. At the onset of infection, which clinically was compatible with glandular fever, there was neutropaenia (WBC total 2,550 and 50 per cent

lymphocytes, some of which were atypical), and relative lympho-
cytosis. No titre of heterophil antibody was reported. Seven weeks
later, when his white-cell count was 8,000 and the blood smear was
'returning to normal', he complained of sudden tinnitus and labyrinthine symptoms. (Eleven days previously he had had oral type III
polio vaccine, a virus not then reported as affecting the labyrinth.)
The evidence in this paper is not convincing in support of the
authors' claim, nor were they able to find other cases in the literature.

Whetnall (1964) considered it a probable cause of perceptive deafness in two children.

More recently it has been recognised that patients who have had
glandular fever have antibody in their sera to the Epstein–Barr
virus, which is considered transmissible in saliva. This suggests that
the virus is the aetiological agent in glandular fever.

Measles

Lindsay and Hemenway (1954) described the case of deafness following measles in a seven months old child a few weeks previously.
The histopathology included subacute inflammatory changes in the
cochlea, saccule, utricle and canals. This case showed extruded cells
on the surface of the stria vascularis, including lymphocytes, and
monocytes and giant cells were seen in the fluid of the cochlear
canal. There were papillomatous lesions in the wall of the utricle.

Nager's (1907) cases lived three years after measles at the age of
three. The tectorial membrane was rolled up, and covered by
flattened cells in the basal coil, which was the only part of the
cochlea to show degeneration of peripheral nerve fibres and ganglion cells. The utricle and saccule were dilated, as was the cochlear
duct of the basal cochlear turn.

Lindsay and Hemenway (1954) refer to a third case in the literature, where a bacterial meningitis had supervened.

Lindsay (1967) comments that of the cases so far described, the
1954 case is the only sub-acute one, where inflammatory changes
are still to be seen.

Beal, Davey and Lindsay (1967a) described the pathology of a
case of possible acquired deafness due to measles at sixteen months,
on a congenital Mondini type of abnormality. The same authors

(1967b) and Hemenway describe two cases of suddenly acquired deafness in adults following viral infection in one case, and an unknown immediate past history in the other. Histopathology in both patients was that described for mumps, measles and rubella.

Mumps

Deafness as a complication of mumps was noted by Hippocrates, whose account of the disease is quoted in Major's *Classic Descriptions*.

A histopathological description by Lindsay, Davey and Ward (1960) shows that there was degeneration of the cochlear duct and the structures in it, with a mild degree of degeneration of the spiral ganglion in the basal coil. There was severe bilateral damage coming on three weeks after the onset of mumps. The patient was a 5 year old boy, who developed haematuria. The cause of death, within the next year, was 'inclusion cell encephalitis', which was also given as the cause in Lindsay and Hemenway's case of measles (1954).

There was marked strial atrophy; the tectorial membrane was rolled up and covered by a cellular layer in the apical coil, and probably absent in the basal coil. The organ of Corti was absent.

Prasad's (1963) case of bilateral deafness in mumps is interesting because the author investigated the cerebrospinal fluid and found sixty-two white cells per cubic millimetre (all lymphocytes), without abnormality. The onset of labyrinthine symptoms occured fourteen days after the clinical diagnosis of mumps.

Bocca and Giordano (1956) investigated twenty-eight cases of sudden deafness thought to be due to eighth nerve neuronitis. Some cases, considered to be due to mumps, have recovered (Harbert and Young, 1964).

Van Dishoeck and Bierman (1957) found mumps a cause of about two-thirds of the (twenty-two) cases of neuronitis considered to have a viral aetiology when they investigated sixty-six cases of sudden deafness.

Schuknecht *et al.* (1962) conclude that mumps virus has an important role in the aetiology of sudden deafness. They describe the pathology of four cases. Mumps as a cause of multiple embryopathy has also been recognised (*Lancet*, 1966).

Cytomegalic inclusion disease

Inclusion-bearing cells have been recognised in infants, either in salivary gland epithelial cells or in generalised, usually epithelial, distribution of the disseminated form, which has been estimated as occurring in less than 2 per cent of infant autopsies (Wyatt *et al.*, 1956). As the infant clinical syndrome may be thrombocytopenic purpura, haemolytic anaemia, pneumonitis and cerebral calcifications, this virus disease enters into the differential diagnosis of the 'generalised rubella syndrome', and of toxoplasmosis, and disseminated herpes virus infection.

In adults the disease has been described in those who were debilitated, on cytotoxic drugs, steroids or dying of other disease. Symmers (1960) has described it as an 'opportunistic' disease. It may be that it has remained latent throughout life. It may also be acquired, usually in the course of multiple blood transfusions such as would be required for cardiac surgery. Histological evidence of infection comes from finding the characteristic inclusions in cells —not so commonly in the epithelial cells—as in infants, but in the endothelial cells of the blood vessels. Ward *et al.* (1965) identified it in the vascular endothelium of the laryngeal surface of the epiglottis, and in vascular endothelium in a small vessel in the petrous apex, in a woman dying of ulcerative colitis and disseminated sclerosis. They refer to an earlier identification in tissue from an acute mastoiditis, by Symmers (1960), in a woman of 34 who died of Wegener's granulomatosis.

Hanshaw (1966), in a comprehensive review of the literature on the virus and the congenital and acquired forms of the disease it causes, refers to eighteen infants from whom cytomegalovirus was isolated in Rochester, N.Y., during the first twelve months of life. Thirteen of the infants were 'adequately observed' for neurological sequelae, and one of them was deaf. Other series with descriptions of neurological involvement make no mention of hearing loss, but this may be an omission of examination at the right age. The case discussed by Hanshaw was born weighing 6 lb 1 oz at term to a 17 year old primigravida. At nine weeks she had a whooping-cough-like illness and a white-cell count of 12,150 (80 per cent lymphocytes). Culture for Bordetella pertussis was negative, but the CFT for cytomegalovirus was positive at a titre of 1/64, and subsequently the virus was isolated from the throat and urine. She had persistent viruria till twelve months of age. At forty months of age she was referred to the Rochester School for the Deaf as 'speech and language retardation probably based on mental retardation of unknown aetiology'. She did not respond to environmental sound of at least 60 dB SPL.

Varicella-zoster virus

This is a DNA virus, and is classed with the Papova viruses.

Papilloma and wart viruses, 40–55 millimicrons.

Adenoviruses, 65–87 millimicrons.

Herpes virus, 120–180 millimicrons.

Pox viruses, 150–300 millimicrons.

The herpes group also includes cytomegalovirus.

Acquired Varicella-zoster virus is identified as icosahedral in shape in its intracellular form; the capsid includes 162 hollow capsomeres (Almeida *et al.*, 1962). The size of the mature form is 200 millimicrons. The capsomere is protein, with protein coats. The virus must attach to the wall of a host cell before it can penetrate. The cell then phagocytoses the virus: the virus reaches the nucleus, where it multiplies, making use of the replicating nuclear activity of the host cell. It gathers the requisite protein coats also from the host cell, as it passes out of the cell.

Once in the cell, phospholipids are removed by a digestion process, leaving the virus DNA unrepressed, and messenger RNA and ribosomes make an uncoating protein, which, in two hours or less in tissue culture, removes the last protective layer, leaving the viral DNA naked, in which state it is free to go to work. The viral genome now enters the nucleus and takes over the host genetic apparatus. If the cell multiplies, so does the virus: if not, the virus must remain dormant and hence uninfective.

The epidemiological cycle of this virus has been investigated and discussed by Hope-Simpson (1965). The latent virus, after an attack of varicella, remains dormant in the cells of the dorsal root ganglion and possibly elsewhere in the nervous system; the cells do not divide, hence the virus cannot do so. If the virus did, and was released, postvaricellar neutralising antibodies would inhibit its infecting other cells. In old age, and debility of all sorts, with cytotoxic drugs and with x-rays, ability to maintain the titre of antibody falls. If at the same time the host cells are damaged, and viral infective particles released, then a typical zoster rash and neuritis appear.

Unlike spinal zoster, cephalic zoster (a useful term we owe to Rebattu, Mounier-Kuhn *et al.*, 1933) involves one or more cranial nerves. The raised lymphocyte count and protein in the cerebrospinal fluid suggests that all zoster is really an encephalomyelitis (Rose *et al.*, 1964) and that the brain stem and cervical cord at least are involved.

Auditory nerve damage in zoster is uncommon: it is probably commonest in the form associated with facial nerve palsy. Blackley *et al.* (1967) have agreed this is a more complicated disease than Ramsay Hunt's concept of geniculate ganglionitis would indicate: the temporal bone of the affected side of the case described by them showed intense perivascular, perineural and intraneural round cell aggregations, also in the cochlea and the mastoid process, and beneath the skin, seven months after the eruption of the rash. Hope-Simpson states that seventh and eighth nerve palsy occurs in three to four cases per thousand of population per year. It is possible that 'auditory zoster' may occur without a rash, as Phillips (1963) has claimed, and if so it may account for some sudden-onset cases of deafness. Rebattu *et al.* (1933) found eighty-two cases where eighth nerve involvement was studied: only 11 per cent showed vestibular involvement alone, 45 per cent cochlear only; in the remaining 44 per cent both branches were involved.

The pathology of the cochlea in the case described by Blackley *et al.* included opacity of the endolymph and perilymph, suggesting high protein content. There was lymphocytic infiltration beneath the stria vascularis and in the spiral ligament. Reissner's membrane had collapsed in all turns, and the destruction of the organ of Corti was most complete in the apical turn. This description, which is of the third temporal bone to be sectioned whole from this condition, resembles the results of a neuronitis rather than a primary lesion in the stria vascularis as is seen in many viral diseases.

Congenital: deafness following maternal varicella-zoster Laforet and Lynch (1947) reported a case of multiple congenital abnormalities in a new-born baby whose mother had had varicella in the eighth week of pregnancy. These were mainly defects of the central nervous system and one lower limb: the infant had bilateral optic atrophy, and appears to have survived at any rate to the age of six months. They refer to a case where the mother produced a 'healthy infant' after varicella in the second week of pregnancy. (It is not implied that deafness was excluded.) They give several references to cases of congenital varicella where an infant is born with the eruption or develops it very soon after birth, and drew the distinction between this and a case early in pregnancy which might result in defective development.

It is clear, however, that damage to this foetus may resemble that of maternal rubella, for three of the four cases referred to by Lamy *et al.* (1951) had deafness and a cardiac defect, accompanied by pseudoretinitis pigmentosa (Laplane, Bregeat and Ossipovski, no reference given: no further details quoted). Duehr (1955) reports two cases of congenital cataract in children whose mothers had typical herpes zoster during early pregnancy, one probably in the fourth month and the other during the third month.

The second case also had microphthalmos: the first, mental retardation and talipes equinovarus. Bradford Hill *et al.* (1958) concluded that chickenpox carried a risk of low birth weight rather than malformation. Michon *et al.* (1959) have reported two cases following zoster in the seventh to ninth weeks and the second month respectively. These cases showed central nervous system and skeletal deformities. Wilson (1960) reports a healthy infant following maternal zoster at four months. Maran (1966) mentions a case of acquired sensorineural deafness which preceded the varicellar eruption in a 16 year old girl, but no case of congenital deafness due to this virus. It may be that damage can occur, during the viraemia, and that foetal embryopathy is to be expected where maternal antibody is low as is likely in zoster. Neither disease is commonest in the child-bearing years, which may account for the scarcity of cases.

Rubella

Gregg (1941) observed that maternal rubella during the first trimester of pregnancy could produce congenital cataract. This observation was made during the Australian epidemic of 1939–40, which was both virulent and widespread, as the disease had not occurred in epidemic form for seventeen years, and thus a whole generation was susceptible. Swan and Tostevin (1946) added microcephaly, deafness and congenital heart disease to the syndrome.

The risk to the foetus was over-estimated at first, being subject to the slant of all retrospective surveys. Lundstrom (1962) and Manson *et al.* (1960), using the prospective method of follow-ups of children born of rubella-affected pregnancies, estimated the incidence of major defects as shown in table VIII.

Table VIII Rubella in months of pregnancy

Month:	1	2	3	4	5+	Controls
Lundstrom						
Defects/cases	13/117	18/157	15/189	3/209	2/474	5/712
Per cent	11	11·5	7·9	1·5	0·4	0·7
Manson *et al.*						
Defects/cases	7/45	12/61	10/77	3/72	5/288	128/5,455
Per cent	15·6	19·7	13	4·2	1·7	2·3

The clinical diagnosis of the disease is not always easy, and until Parkman *et al.* (1962) and Weller and Neva (1962) developed tissue culture techniques the rubella virus was uncultivable. It is possible to establish the presence of the virus in the pharynx and in the blood at the time of enlargement of occipital lymph nodes. Seven or eight days later (the sixteenth day from infection) the maculopapular rash appears, the virus disappears from the blood, neutralising antibody appears and increases. After another eight days the pharynx and intestine are usually free of virus. It may be excreted in the urine for longer. Heggie (1966) discusses the epidemiology and teratology.

The transmission across the placenta and persistence of the virus Rubella virus was recovered from an embryo aborted ten days after maternal rubella (Selzer, 1963). Heggie and Weir (1964) noted that viral persistence in a similar case is much longer than in post-natal-acquired rubella. Alford *et al.* (1964) noted extreme chronicity of infection, which was still present several weeks after birth.

Phillips *et al.* (1965) followed up eighty-five infants whose mothers had had rubella during the first three months of pregnancy: some had congenital defects, others were clinically normal. Thirty-two per cent had rubella virus in the throat during the first month of life,

15 per cent in the third: the percentages for urine and faeces also fell from 19 and 12 per cent to 6 and 3 per cent. Horstmann (1965) recovered rubella virus from the pharynx of infants which had clinical evidence of rubella syndrome in higher percentages. These also fell with the passage of time: eighty-two per cent were positive at birth, 50 per cent in the third month, and none after the ninth month. These infants are of course contagious.

Recovery of virus from abortions for maternal rubella is high, probably 40–60 per cent (Alford et al., 1964). Spontaneous abortions occur in 10–15 per cent of pregnancies affected by rubella (Tartakov, 1965, and others). There is the possibility that some of the curettage specimens are evidence of placental infection only, not necessarily of foetal infections.

Antibodies in the infant Rubella-neutralising antibody has been detected in clinically affected infants at birth, and also in the un-infected infant whose mother has neutralising antibody (Alford et al., 1964, and others). The antibody of the uninfected infant declines (Dudgeon et al., 1964), persisting only in the congenitally affected.

The congenital rubella syndrome Dent et al. (1968) explain the paradox of persistent virus excretion by an infant which has circulating 19S antibodies, and who should thus be immune. As immune response is provoked by the virus, and thus 'tolerance' is not present, these authors suggest that a defect in cellular immune functions has occurred. They failed *in vitro* to demonstrate cellular anti-viral activity. The rubella-infection of the human lymphocyte appears to produce inability to complete the cellular metabolic changes required for full immunological functions.

The pathology of the cochlea in congenital rubella This somewhat resembles the strial lesion of adult mumps: a proliferative granulomatous lesion can be seen in affected cases (Friedmann and Wright, 1966). In a further case in a child of six months with the congenital rubella syndrome, the main points of the pathology were the degeneration of the organ of Corti, presumably secondary to the vascular lesion in the stria, and thus compatible with previously normal maturation of the neuroepithelial cells. The tectorial membrane, as in mumps and measles, was shrivelled and had a cellular covering, and Reissner's membrane was partially collapsed.

Other cases of rubella deafness in which the histopathology of the cochlea is described are Carruthers (1945), Lindsay *et al.* (1953), Schall *et al.* (1951), Kelemen and Gotlib (1959), Ward, Honrubia and Moore (1968), and Kelemen (1966).

Histopathology of other aspects of rubella infection is described by Plotkin, Oski *et al.* (1965) and in human embryo tissue culture by Plotkin, Boue and Boue (1965). Plotkin (1964) isolated rubella virus from patients with thrombocytopaenic purpura.

Menser *et al.* (1967c) reviewed the congenital rubella syndrome as a whole in a twenty-five year follow-up, and reported (1967a) renal arterial intimal proliferation in infants, and (1967b) persistence of rubella virus in the lens. Nusbacher *et al.* (1967) have shown that chromosomes from affected foetuses have more than the expected number of abnormalities.

A prospective survey

Other possible intra-uterine virus diseases causing congenital defects were investigated by means of a prospective survey following up the offspring of about 12,000 women who were investigated between April 1959 and the end of 1960 in Great Britain. Ninety-five per cent were available for follow-up and eighty-eight per cent at the end of the second year of life. The results were (McDonald, personal communication, 1968):

2·1 per cent: pregnancies ended in abortion.
1·8 per cent: pregnancies ended in still birth.
4·7 per cent: a major congenital defect.
11·5 per cent: a minor defect.

Some relationship was found with febrile respiratory illness during the first eight weeks of pregnancy.

References

Alford, C.A., Neva, F.A., Weller, T.H. (1964), *New Eng. J. Med. 271*, 1275.
Almeida, J.D., Howartson, A.F., and Williams, M.G. (1962), *Virology, 16*, 353.

Beal, D.D., Davey, P.R., and Lindsay, J. (1967a), *Arch. Otolaryng.* 85, 134.

Beal, D.D., Hemenway, W.G., and Lindsay, J.R. (1967b) *Arch. Otolaryng.* 85, 591.

Blackley, B., Friedmann, I., and Wright, I. (1967), *Acta Otolaryng.* 63, 533.

Bocca, E., and Giordano, R. (1956), *Arch. Ital. Otol.* 67, 70.

Bradford Hill, A., Doll, R., Galloway, T.McL., and Hughes, J.P.W. (1958), *Brit. Jl. Prev. Soc. Med.* 12, 1.

Carruthers, D.G. (1945), *Med. J. Aust.* 1, 315.

Chanock, R.M., Parrot, R.H., Vargosko, A.J., Kapikian, A.Z., Kugurt, V., and Johnson, K.H. (1962), *Amer. J. Publ. Health*, 52, 918.

Chanock, R.M., and Parott, R.H. (1965), *Pediatrics* (Springfield, Ill.), 36, 21.

Currie, J.A. (1961), *Proc. Roy. Soc. Med.* 54, 290.

Dawes, J.D.K. (1951), 'Myringitis bullosa haemorrhagica: its relationship to encephalitis and cranial nerve paralyses', unpublished M.D. thesis, Durham.

— (1953), *J. Laryng.* 67, 313.

— (1963), *Proc. Roy. Soc. Med.* 56, 777.

Dent, P.B., Olson, G.B., Good, R.A., Rawls, W.E., South, M.A., and Melnick, J.L. (1968), *Lancet*, 1, 291.

Dudgeon, J.A., Butler, N.R., and Plotkin, S.A. (1964), *Brit. Med. Jl.* 2, 155.

Duehr, P. (1955) *Am. J. Ophth.* 39, 157.

Epstein, M.A., Henle, G., Achong, B.G., and Barr, M. (1965), *J. Exp. Med.* 121, 761.

Falconer, J. (1852), *Annals of Influenza*, p. 254, Sydenham Society, London.

Friedmann, I., and Wright, I. (1966), *Brit Med. Jl.* 2, 20.

Gregg, J.B., and Shaeffer, J.H. (1964), *South Dakota Jl. Med. Pharm.* 17, 22.

Gregg, N.McA. (1941), *Tr. Ophth. Soc. Austral.* 3, 35.

Hanshaw, J.B. (1966), *Ped. Clin. of N. America*, 13, 279.

Harbert, F., and Young, I.M. (1964), *Arch. Otolaryng.* 79, 459.

Heggie, A.D., and Weir, W.C. (1964), *Pediatrics*, 34, 278.

Heggie, A.D. (1966), *N. Ped. Clin. N. Amer.* 13, 251.

Hers, J.F.Ph., Masurel, N., and Mulder, J. (1958), *Lancet*, 2, 1141.

Hilleman, M.R., and Werner, J.H. (1954), *Proc. Soc. Exp. Biol.* (N.Y.), 85, 183.

Hope-Simpson, R.E. (1965), *Proc. Roy. Soc. Med.* 58, 9.

Horstmann, D.M. (1965), *California Med.* 102, 397.

James, T. (1964), *S. Afric. Med. Jl. 38*, 709.

Keleman, G., and Gotlib, B.N. (1959), *Laryngoscope, 69*, 385.

Kelemen, G. (1966), *Arch. Otolaryng. 83*, 520.

Kuroya, M., Ishida, N., and Shiratori, T. (1953), *Yokohama Med. Bull. 4*, 217.

Laforet, E.G., and Lynch, C.L. (1947), *New Eng. J. Med. 236*, 534.

Lamy, M., Minkowski, A., and Choucroun, J. (1951), 'Semaine médicale', supp. to *Semaine des hôpitaux, 27*, 989.

Leading article, *The Lancet* (1952), *1*, 299.

Leading article, *The Lancet* (1966), *2*, 692.

Lindsay, J.R. (1967), *Acta Otolaryng. 63*, 138.

Lindsay, J.R., Davey, P.R., and Ward, P.H. (1960), *Ann. Otol. 69*, 918.

Lindsay, J.R., Carruthers, D.G., Hemenway, W.G., and Harrison, S. (1953), *Ann. Otol. 62*, 1201.

Lindsay, J.R., and Hemenway, W.G. (1954), *Ann. Otol. 63*, 754.

Lundstrom, R. (1962), *Acta paed. 51*, supp., 133.

Manson, M.M., Logan, W.P.D., and Loy, R.M. (1960), *Reports on the Public Health and Medical Subjects*, No. 101, Ministry of Health, H.M.S.O., London.

McDonald, J.C. (1968), personal communication, to be published.

Maran, A.C. (1966), *J. Laryng. 80*, 495.

Marshall, J.B. (1955), *Lancet, 1*, 458.

Menser, M.A., Dods, L., and Harley, J.D. (1967a), *Lancet, 1*, 571.

— (1967b), *Lancet, 2*, 771.

— (1967c), *Lancet, 2*, 1347.

Michon, L., Aubertin, D., and Jager-Schmidt, G. (1959), *Arch. Franc. Pediat. 16*, 695.

Miller, H.G., Stanton, J.B., and Gibbons, J.L. (1956), *Quart. J. Med. 25*, 427; (1957) *Brit. Med. Jl. i*, 668.

Morris, J.A., Blount, R.E., Jr. and Savage, R.E. (1956), *Proc. Soc. Exp. Biol.* (N.Y.), *92*, 544.

Nager, F.R. (1907), *Z. Ohrenheilk. 54*, 217.

Newell Price, J.C. (1956), *Research Newsletter* of Coll. Gen. Pract., referred to by Currie.

Nusbacher, J., Hirschhorn, K., and Cooper, L.Z. (1967), *New Eng. J. Med. 276*, 1409.

Parkmann, P.D., Buescher, E.L., and Altenstein, M.S. (1962), *Proc. Soc. Exp. Biol.* (N.Y.), *111*, 225.

Pedersen, E. (1959), *Brain, 82*, 566.

Phillips, B.L.D. (1963), *British J. Clin. Pract. 17*, 715.

Phillips, C.A., Melnick, J.L., Yow, M.D., Bayatpour, M., and Burkharat, M. (1965), *J. Amer. Med. Assn. 193*, 1027.

Plotkin, S.A. (1964), *J. Amer. Med. Assn. 190*, 265.
Plotkin, S.A., Oski, F.A., Hartnett, E.M., Hervada, A.R., Friedman, S., and Gowing, J. (1965), *J. Paediatr. 67*, 182.
Plotkin, S.A., Boue, A., and Boue, G. (1965), *Am. J. Epid. 81*, 71.
Prasad, L.N. (1963), *J. Laryng. 77*, 809.
Price, W.H. (1956), *Proc. Nat. Acad. Sci.* (Washington, D.C.), *42*, 892.
Rebattu, J., Mounier-Kuhn, P., Dechaume, J., Bonnet, P., and Colrat, A. (1933), *Rev. d'oto-neuro-opht. 11*, 241–406.
Rifkind, D., Chanock, R., Kravetz, H., Johnson, K., and Knight, V. (1962), *Am. Rev. Resp. Dis. 85*, 479.
Rose, F.C., Brett, E.M., and Burston, J. (1964), *Arch. Neurol.* (Chicago), *11*, 155.
Rowe, W.P., Huebner, R.J.G., Gilmore, L.K., Parrott, R.H., and Ward, T.G. (1953), *Proc. Soc. Exp. Biol.* (N.Y.), *84*, 570.
Sataloff, J., and Vasallo, L. (1968), *Arch. Otolaryng. 87*, 74.
Schall, L.A., Lurie, M.H., and Kelemen, G. (1951), *Laryngoscope, 61*, 99.
Schuknecht, H.F., Benitez, J., Beckhuis, J., Igarashi, M., Singleton, G., and Rüedi, L. (1962), *Laryngoscope, 72*, 1142.
Selzer, G. (1963), *Lancet, 2*, 336.
Stuart-Harris, C.H. (1963), *J. Laryng. 77*, 979.
Swan, C., and Tostevin, A.L. (1946), *Med. J. Austral. 1*, 645.
Symmers, W.StC. (1960), *J. Clin. Path. 13*, 1.
Tartakov, I.J. (1965), *J. Pediatr. 66*, 380.
Tilles, J.G., Klein, J.O., Jao, R.L., Haslam, J.E., Feingold, M., Gellis, S.S., and Finland, M. (1967), *New Eng. J. Med. 277*, 613.
Tóth, M., Barna, M., and Voltai, B. (1965), *Acta Paediatr. Acad. Sci. Hung. 6*, 367.
Tyrell, D.J., and Parsons, R. (1960), *Lancet, 1*, 239.
Van Dishoeck, H.A.E., and Bierman, T.A. (1957), *Ann. Otol. 66*, 963.
Ward, P.H., Lindsay, J.R., and Warner, N.E. (1965), *Laryngoscope, 75*, 628.
Ward, P.H., Honrubia, V., and Moore, B.S. (1968), *Arch. Otolaryng. 87*, 22.
Weller, T.H., and Neva, F.A. (1962), *Proc. Soc. Exp. Biol.* (N.Y.), *111*, 215.
Whetnall, E., and Fry, D.B. (1964), *The Deaf Child*, Heinemann, London.
Wilson, E. (1960), *Med. J. Austral. 2*, 63.
Wyatt, J.P., Saxton, J., Lee, R.S., and Pinkerton, H. (1950), *J. Pediatr. 36*, 271.

XVIII Syphilis

The causative organism of syphilis is *Treponema pallidum*. It is an uncultivable organism: Noguchi's anaerobic cultures are generally regarded as non-pathogenic, at least within a few years' subculture. It is protozoal, motile, a spiral organism which is difficult to stain (hence 'pallidum'). Survival times in strict anaerobiosis are usually less than twenty hours. Attempts at tissue culture of this organism using HeLa, human amnion, rabbit testis and rabbit kidney cells have failed (Wright, 1962), though attachment of motile forms to monolayer cells could be demonstrated under dark-field illumination. No penetration of cells was identified. Electron microscopy has revealed an interesting structure (Ovcinnikov and Delectorski, 1965, 1968) but has cast no light on the method of cell multiplication. Inoculation of chick otocyst in aerobic conditions and in anti-biotic-free medium resulted in apparent penetration of a nerve fibre by *T. pallidum* (Wright and Bird, unpublished).

The organism may be acquired sexually or non-sexually, or as a congenital infection across the placenta.

Acquired syphilis

The pathology of acquired syphilitic causation of deafness is somewhat obscure. Two main types of nervous-system syphilis occur: both are in the tertiary stage of the disease, which may become manifest within few or many years of infection.

Meningovascular or cerebrospinal syphilis is essentially a lesion of the blood vessels: there is endarteritic thickening and perivascular inflammation, infiltrating the perivascular space. This impairs the blood supply to the tissues, thrombosis may occur, and hence areas of necrosis and caseation may be found. This response is a granuloma, surrounded by fibrotic tissue, and is the equivalent of a gumma anywhere else: it is rarely large in the central nervous system.

Parenchymatous syphilis has usually no vascular disturbance in the nervous system. Atrophy occurs of the dorsal and spinal roots and dorsal columns; microscopically the lesion is a demyelination of the affected fibres producing *Tabes dorsalis*. There is secondary neuroglial proliferation, with overlying thickening of the pia mater. Brain considered that no theory of the selectivity of the spinal cord lesions was satisfactory. The second form of parenchymatous syphilis is general paresis in which the anterior cerebral hemispheres are shrunken, with secondary hydrocephalus. The leptomeninges show round-cell infiltration, also particularly seen in the perivascular spaces of the cortex. Ganglion cells degenerate.

The cranial nerves may be affected, as in optic atrophy and the Argyll–Robertson pupil in tabes. It is likely that these lesions may be mediated through the pathology of meningovascular disease. Merritt, Adams and Solomon (1964) found that the eighth nerve, auditory or vestibular division, was next most likely to be involved in tabes: 28 per cent of their tabetic patients had hearing impairment, but they regarded the syphilitic causation as obscure. They found auditory nerve involvement in cases of meningeal neurosyphilis; this is an early manifestation of syphilis, usually within the first two years of infection, and includes syphilitic hydrocephalus (twenty-eight cases, no cranial nerve lesions), meningitis of the vertex (twenty cases, two with cranial nerve involvement, one of which had bilateral deafness, but interestingly, no facial nerve palsy), and basal syphilitic meningitis (thirty-four cases, all with multiple cranial nerve involvement, fourteen with eighth nerve involvement and four of these bilateral).

Budd (1842) remarked that focal neurological signs in a young person should suggest syphilis: in 1847, Virchow confirmed this in his paper on syphilitic arterial inflammation, and Huebner (1874) appreciated that most cerebral syphilitic clinical lesions stem from disease of the blood vessels. Merritt, Adams and Solomon found three cases of eighth nerve involvement out of forty-two cases of cerebrovascular syphilis.

In fact, neurologists tend to regard syphilitic sensorineural deafness as neuronal, rather than due to end-organ changes.

When we turn to the histopathology of the middle ear and of the cochlea there is some reason for confusion. As late as 1928 Alexander demonstrated a belief in the syphilitic causation of otosclerosis, and hence some of his conclusions may be disregarded. Nevertheless he illustrates a lesion which he attributes to syphilitic bone disease of the middle ear, with vascular shunts. Eggston and Wolff illustrate ossification of the ampulla of the posterior semi-circular canal, and fracture of the otic capsule, in a case of acquired syphilis: new bone was also seen in part of the vestibule. Perilymphatic fibrosis and bone formation has been seen in the semi-circular canals by Good-hill (1939), and by Mayer and Fraser (1936), and it is of course accepted that two of the manifestations of syphilis are periostitis and osteomyelitis. Goodhill, who also reviews the early literature, compares acquired and congenital cases, describing the pathology in twenty-six temporal bones. Both groups showed:

1. 'Non-gummatous' productive periostitis, involving the semi-circular canals particularly, and the ductus endolymphaticus in one case.
2. A deformity of the stapedial foot-plate (which appears to be possibly due to the angle of sectioning).
3. Atrophy of the organ of Corti. The spiral ganglion cells were seen variably but frequently.
4. Round-cell infiltration in the cochlea, along the basement membrane and in the stria vascularis, in the spiral ligament, and also of the fibres of the eighth nerve.
5. Vascular changes of an obliterative nature.

No changes suggestive of gummata were seen in the otic capsule, other than round-cell infiltration, though Mayer and Fraser demonstrate the miliary gumma in the stria vascularis.

Alergant (1965) described an eighth nerve lesion in early syphilis, describing it as a rarely encountered type of case. It was considered to be a secondary syphilitic manifestation. Moore (1947), on the other hand, considers an eighth nerve lesion early in syphilis to be always due to acute syphilitic meningitis.

Grünberg's (1910) case (a young man of 21 years who had acquired syphilis two years earlier) showed similar changes to those in the acquired cases of Goodhill's. Clinically, the case had gummatous changes in the nasopharynx, so might be considered as a tertiary case or late secondary.

An attempt at experimental simulation of middle-ear infection with *T. pallidum* suspension has failed to produce more than early inflammation of the bulla after six days in guinea-pigs (Wright, unpublished). This animal is held to be intermediate in susceptibility between the rabbit and man: inoculation produces little local response, but on intra-testicular inoculation quickly becomes a generalised infection (Willcox and Guthe, 1966).

The inoculation of a chick otocyst with an active suspension of *T. pallidum* showed that some penetration of the tissue had occurred, and one treponeme was seen apparently in a nerve fibre.

Congenital syphilis

Pathology The characteristic history of a family produced by syphilitic parents is one of severe congenital disease, resulting in abortions, followed by less severe disease, resulting in still-births, and ultimately—presumably as maternal antibody titres remained protective but the likelihood of parasitaemia became less—the births of living children, in whom the stigmata of congenital syphilis would be found, such as the saddle-nose. Later still those with healthy infancies might yet develop the 'Hutchinsonian' triad of peg-shaped, notched upper incisors, interstitial keratitis, and perceptive deafness.

In spite of failure to cultivate in its pathogenic state, considerable knowledge has been acquired of the natural history of *T. pallidum* in animals (Turner and Hollander, 1957; Willcox and Guthe, 1966), its immunology in animals and man, and the histopathology of the disease it produces (WHO technical report, 1970).

The placenta is chiefly affected in congenital syphilis, except perhaps in late post-conceptional syphilitic infection (MacCallum, 1940). There is a marked enlargement of the placenta, which shows bulbous swelling of the villi due to vascular intimal and adventitial thickening, considerable infiltration by wandering cells, and formation of loose connective tissue about the central blood vessels. Similar changes are seen in the umbilical cord. The spirochaete enters the foetal tissues and multiplies to an extent never found in adult acquired syphilis. It is found in astounding numbers, when a silver stain is used, lying between the cells without producing much evident change. MacCallum considers this may be due to the death of the infant *in utero*, perhaps with an interval of some days before a specimen is taken for histological examination, the dead tissue providing an ideal culture medium which is non-resistant and at a suitable temperature. The babies showing the most extreme lesions are not particularly those in whose tissues abundant spirochaetes are found.

MacCallum states that lesions due to the spirochaete are impossible to demonstrate earlier than the fifth month. As a blood-borne infection, generalised tissue destruction may occur, with later scarring. There may be retardation and distortion, well seen in the development of the long bones. The lungs are heavily infiltrated with white cells and histiocytes and increased connective tissue ('pneumonia alba'). There is widespread periostitis and perichondritis: ulceration in the nasal passages leads to snuffles. The liver has a pericellular fibrosis, and may still be the site of extramedullary haemopoiesis. The pancreas is also affected.

Syphilitic osteochondritis is most developed in the epiphyseal region at the knee.

Later forms show gummatous destruction, e.g. the saddle nose, bossing of the frontal bones, and generally dwarfing. All the late forms of acquired syphilis—e.g. Clutton's joints, tabes, general paresis—have been recorded following the congenital disease.

An early (1861) clinical lecture on congenital syphilis by Hutchinson underlines the importance of the notched, peg-shaped upper incisors in diagnosing the condition. (This is to be found in Major's *Classic Descriptions of Disease* and in the reference below). There is a detailed description of the teeth but no mention of deafness, the significance of which Hutchinson had evidently not then seen. The cases described were of the severer sort: eldest living children of their parents. This clinical lecture also includes Hutchinson's technique for eliciting confirmatory history without arousing the suspicions of the mother and thus 'arousing family mistrust'.

The still-birth or young infant severely afflicted with syphilis is likely to exhibit syphilitic pathology in the middle ear and cochlea. Grünberg's (1911) case with spirochaetes within the vessels in the temporal bone was of this variety. If an infant survives and is found to have the early form of syphilitic deafness, it will have meningoneuritis, meningoneurolabyrinthitis or otolabyrinthitis.

The 'late form' of syphilitic hearing loss   In 1863 Hutchinson described the late-onset sensorineural hearing loss due to congenital

syphilis and associated with interstitial keratitis and 'peg-top' upper
incisor teeth. Hutchinson found that twenty-three of the 122 cases
of congenital syphilis seen by him at the Hospital for Sick Children
had a hearing defect. Few of these cases were followed into adult
life, so that the actual prevalence is probably much higher (Nabarro,
1954). Recently Karmody and Schuknecht (1966) stated that
38 per cent of a series of 122 congenital syphilitics treated at the
Massachusetts General Hospital between 1942 and 1964 had a
hearing loss. These authors also consider that the actual prevalence
is likely to be higher because some cases were followed for a few
years only. Dalsgaard–Nielsen (1938) described cases of this type
of hearing loss in the older age groups. She followed 173 patients
with interstitial keratitis and found that the age of onset of the
hearing loss, which occurred in twenty-seven patients, was as
follows: five for age 8–10 years; ten for age 11–20 years; three for
age 21–30 years; four for age 31–40 years; two for age 41–50 years
and three for age 51–60 years.

In order to establish the prevalence, age of onset and relation to
treatment of this type of hearing loss, it would seem worthwhile to
investigate patients with sensorineural hearing loss who could be
shown to have treponemal antibodies in their serum. Modern specific
serological methods show a high degree of certainty as regards
aetiology. Although Mayer and Fraser (1936) and earlier authors
had to accept that this form of hearing loss was compatible with
negative tests for syphilis, today this is not so. Since the use of
new tests, a number of patients who would otherwise have been
regarded as suffering from sensorineural hearing loss of unknown
aetiology have in fact recalled a history of treatment for congenital
syphilis many years previously.

In London in 1962–66, 3 per cent of cases of sensorineural deafness attending the Royal National Throat, Nose and Ear Hospital
were due to congenital syphilis. A further 2 per cent of cases had
either coincidental yaws or acquired syphilis. Some of the congenital cases had received treatment earlier in life, some partial or
even inadvertent treatment. The *T. pallidum* immobilisation test
was useful where the reagin tests were negative or of low titre.
Most of the cases had developed progressive hearing loss in spite of
treatment; further treatment with penicillin did not improve their

audiograms. There was no serological evidence for an auto-immune process (Wright, 1966).

The histopathology of the condition in the ear is somewhat obscure, as Morton (1955, 1956) points out, although Barlow described gummata on cranial nerves, together with cerebrovascular microscopical changes in congenital syphilitic cases, as long ago as 1878. Karmody and Schuknecht (1966) described the histopathology of one case in which the dominant feature was endolymphatic hydrops secondary to osteitis of the otic capsule. Defects in the bone were filled with connective tissue containing lymphocytes, and there was evidence of similar inflammatory tissue in the membranous labyrinth. Karmody and Schuknecht considered that a process of dilatation and rupture of the membranous labyrinth with mixing of perilymph and endolymph accounted for the variation in hearing loss and the sudden attacks of vertigo. Healing followed, but the process was repeated in spite of adequate antisyphilitic treatment in the case that they described. The histopathology is similar to that described by Fraser and Muir (1917) and Mayer and Fraser (1936).

Since the work of Collart and Durel (1964) the survival of typical and atypical forms of *T. pallidum* in cerebrospinal fluid in many cases of acquired syphilis has been recognised. This may account for a persistent *T. pallidum* immobilisation test even though virulence has been lost. The *Treponema* survived treatment, and Collart and Durel assert that treatment given two years after the disease is acquired will not eradicate the parasite from the cerebrospinal fluid. Lawton Smith and Israel (1967) have isolated treponemes from aqueous humour and CSF in sero-negative patients, some of whom were suffering from virulent treponemal disease. The presence of the parasite in the perilymph at least could hardly be disproved at the present time, though this might not be relevant in congenital cases. Kerr *et al.* (1970) have pointed out possible lines of investigation. They refer to the work of W. Griffin and J. Pulec, who are currently examining inner-ear fluids for treponemes. Grünberg (1911) did not find the parasite within the labyrinthine canals of a syphilitic infant. It is to be hoped that any further histopathology of a labyrinth affected by syphilitic disease will include examination by the fluorescent antibody technique. Pieces of tissue, such as the spiral organ, stria vascularis and the spiral ganglion, would require removal by dissection to avoid the long process of decalcification. Moreover, at the same time, this technique would have the advantage of providing identified portions of the spiral organ for phase-contrast examination as described by Engström *et al.* (1966) and by Bredberg (1967). This technique should determine once and for all whether the hair cells sustain damage which temporal bone sections do not demonstrate adequately.

It is interesting to note that in late-onset congenital syphilis of the eye further deteriorations may occur later on in life. There is an association between the development of glaucoma and interstitial keratitis. Hutchinson (1863) himself noted one case of glaucoma in a man of 24 who had had interstitial keratitis at the age of 6. Reports of this association have not been infrequent since then. Britten and Palmer (1964) investigated ninety-five patients suffering from inactive interstitial keratitis. Two patients with advanced glaucoma were found, and seven others with known glaucoma. Three cases had a satisfactory explanation for the development of late glaucoma, namely the presence of peripheral anterior synechiae caused by the anterior segment inflammatory during the active phase of the interstitial keratitis.

The deterioration of hearing later on in life which was noticeable in the Royal National Throat, Nose and Ear Hospital series (Wright, 1966) may thus be an integral part of congenital syphilis, rather than a somewhat early onset of presbyacusis.

References

Alergant, C.D. (1965), *B. J. Ven. Dis. 41*, 300.
Alexander, G. (1928), *Laryngoscope, 38*, 295.
Barlow, T. (1878), 'Meningitis, arteritis and choroiditis in a child the subject of congenital syphilis', *Trans. Path. Soc. Lond. 28*, 287.
— (1878), 'Gummata on cranial nerves; disease of cerebral arteries, cicatrices of liver in spleen in a case of congenital syphilis', *Trans. Path. Soc. Lond. 28*, 291.
Brain, W.R. (1964), *Clinical Neurology*, second edition, Oxford University Press, London.
Bredberg, G. (1967), 'The human cochlea during development and ageing', *J. Laryng. 81*, 79.
Britten, M.J.A., and Palmer, C.A.L. (1964), *Brit. J. Ophthal. 48*, 181.

Budd, G. (1842), *Lond. Med. Gaz.* 2, 357.
Collart, P., and Durel, P. (1964), 'Presence et persistance des tréponèmes dans le L.C.-R. au cours de la syphilis, expérimentale et humaine, après traitement tardif', *Ann. Dermat. Syph.* (Paris), *91*, 485.
Dalsgaard-Nielsen, E. (1938), *Acta Ophth. 16*, 635.
Eggston, A.E., and Wolff, D. (1947), *Histopathology of the Ear, Nose and Throat*, Williams and Wilkins, Baltimore, Md.
Engström, H., Ades, H.W., and Andersson, A. (1966), *The Structural Pattern of the Organ of Corti*, Almqvist and Wiksell, Stockholm.
Fraser, J.S., and Muir, R. (1917), *J. Laryng. 32*, 8.
Goodhill, V. (1939), *Ann. Otol. 48*, 676.
Grünberg, K. (1910), *Z. Ohrenheilk. 60*, 260.
— (1911), *Z. Ohrenheilk, 63*, 223.
Huebner, O. (1874), *Die Luetische Erkrankung der Hinarterien*, Vogel, Leipzig.
Hutchinson, J. (1861), *Brit. Med. Jl. 1*, 515.
— (1863), *Disease of the Eye and Ear Consequent on Inherited Syphilis*, Churchill, London.
Karmody, C.S., and Schuknecht, H.F. (1966), *Arch. Otolaryng. 83*, 18.
Kerr, A.G., Smyth, G.D.L., and Landau, H.D. (1970), *Arch. Otolaryng. 91*, 474.
Lawton Smith. J., and Israel, C.W. (1967), *A.M.A. Arch. Ophthal. 77*, 474.
MacCallum, F.C., *Textbook of Pathology*, seventh edition, 1940, Saunders, Philadelphia and London.
Major, R.H. (1945), *Classic Descriptions of Disease*, third edition, Thomas, Springfield, Ill.
Mayer, O., and Fraser, J.S. (1936), *J. Laryng. 51*, 683 and 755.
Merritt, H.H., Adams, R.D., and Solomon, H.C. (1964), *Neurosyphilis*, Oxford University Press, New York.
Moore, J.E. (1947), *Penicillin in Syphilis*, Blackwell, Oxford.
Morton, R.S. (1955), *Brit. J. Ven. Dis. 31*, 242.
— (1956), *Brit. J. Ven. Dis. 32*, 162.
Nabarro, D. (1954), *Congenital Syphilis*, Arnold, London.
Ovcinnikov, N.M., and Delectorski, V.V. (1965), WHO/VDT/res. 79.65.
— and — (1968), *Brit. J. Ven. Dis. 44*, 1.
Serpetjian, M., Tissot Gueraz, F., Monier, J.C., and Thirolet, J. (1969), WHO/VDT res. 69.180.
Tuffanelli, D.L. (1966), 'Ageing and false positive reactions for syphilis', *Brit. J. Ven. Dis. 42*, 40.
Turner, T.B., and Hollander, D.H. (1957), *The Biology of the Treponematoses*, WHO monograph No. 35, Geneva.

WHO Technical Report series, No. 455 (p. 74), *Treponematoses Research*, Geneva, 1970.

Willcox, R.R., and Guthe, T. (1966), *Treponema pallidum: a bibliographical review of morphology, culture and survival*, WHO bulletin, supplement to vol. 35, Geneva.

Wright, I. (1962), *Proc. Twelfth Internat. Congress Dermatol.*, Washington, vol. 2, p. 884.

— (1966), *Int. Audiol.* 7, 302.

XIX Toxoplasmosis

Toxoplasma gondii was first described by Nicolle and Manceaux (1908), who identified it in the North African gerbil or gondi. It was later described by Castellani (1914). It is now recognised as widely distributed throughout the vertebrate world. The parasite is a protozoon, about 7×2 microns and slightly crescentic in its proliferative form. When found in cells of a host animal it is seen as a cyst or pseudocyst, binary fission having produced up to many hundreds of toxoplasms within the cyst. The parasite has been examined by electron microscopy and found to have a conoid at the pointed end, with toxonemes streaming back from this, and nucleus, Golgi appartus, mitochondria and endoplasmic reticulum. Sheffield and Melton (1968) have examined its fine structures at various stages of cell division.

The parasite can be grown in tissue culture, in any kind of tissue (Cook and Jacobs, 1958). Superficial resemblance to *Encephalitozoon*, *Besnoita*, *Sarcocystis*, *Leishmania*, etc., has largely been resolved by electron microscopy and serological methods (Fulton, 1967). Encysted forms from animal brains have been shown to retain virulence for at least five years (Lainson, 1959).

Routes of infection

Experimentally, any route is satisfactory—oral, subcutaneous, intra-venous or intra-peritoneal. There is soon a parasitaemia, and eventually the parasite will be found in the cells of the central nervous system, in muscle, and to a lesser extent elsewhere. In these sites the parasites encyst, and less commonly in uterus lining, in endo-metrium as well as muscle, intestinal wall and liver.

Human toxoplasmosis

Its parasitism is highly successful, and for most animals, including man, ill effects do not necessarily follow. Remington *et al.* (1961)

have noted parasitaemia in animals even in the presence of high-titre antibody; these authors (1960) also isolated cysts from the human uterus in patients who had antibody. Hogan *et al.* (1958) have recovered the parasite from the eye of a 20 year old man who was considered to have had congenital infection. The retina is more frequently affected than the choroid (Sabin, 1950). There are strains known to be more virulent than others, and strains isolated from different hosts. Virulence of the parasite may reflect weakness of host resistance: toxoplasmosis may be an opportunistic infection.

Acquired human toxoplasmosis is seen as a clinical disease mainly in two forms: the *acquired*, as a glandular-fever-like cervical lymphadenopathy, with a negative Paul–Bunnell test, and charac-teristic granuloma on section; and the *congenital* form following intra-uterine infection. It is clear from such surveys as Robertson's (1962, 1965) in Lincolnshire that sero-positive reactions may increase in a childhood population as the children grow older even though no obvious illness has occurred. (The high rate of positive dye-test reactors in all parts of the world makes the significance of correla-tion of positive results with any particular clinical disease difficult to interpret.) Many investigators have suspected that insect vectors were responsible for transmission, but no convincing evidence has been found. Meat handlers and fur handlers have been found to have significantly higher dye-test titres than the general population. In Britain antibodies are commoner in rural districts than in the towns, but even in neighbouring districts the rates differ (Beverley, 1956). Siim (1961) has isolated parasites from tonsils, which suggests an oral route of infection in the cervical lymphadenopathy form of the disease.

There are, however, virulent human infections reported after laboratory accidents (Beverley *et al.*, 1955). Only one of the eighteen cases discussed by Rawal (1959) was fatal (Sexton *et al.*, 1953). Rawal's own case followed work with RH strain. Many of the cases are reported without mentioning the strain of the parasite respon-sible. Beattie (1964) states that *T. gondii* from severe fatal infections in man have usually proved highly virulent for experimental animals, whereas strains from lymphadenopathies have failed to produce illness in the experimental animal; strains of low virulence are, however, known to become more virulent on subsequent passage, either in the same host or another (Lainson, 1955a).

Recently human cases of myositis (Chandar *et al.* 1968; Rowland and Greer, 1961) and hepatitis (Vischer *et al.*, 1967) have been reported, in addition to the previously recognised myocarditis and pneumonitis. Biopsies showed *Toxoplasma*-like parasites in the affected tissues, in the liver biopsies, fluorescence microscopy was used to detect the parasites.

Congenital infection   It was formerly assumed that congenital infection could affect the foetus only if the mother acquired acute toxoplasmosis during pregnancy. Many instances are now known of women with low antibodies, or even no antibodies, who have produced infected foetuses.

Werner (1962) mentions possible mechanisms of such infections.

Robertson (1966) has reported a case of a woman with repeated chronic abortion, from whose fourth abortion (sixth pregnancy) *T. gondii* were cultured by inoculation into mice. Her dye-test was negative at a titre of 1/8 on all but one 'dubious' occasion, and Robertson quotes Langer's (1963) four sero-negative patients out of twenty-three with parasites isolated from curettings, menstrual fluids, placenta or foetus. Nor is the situation unknown in animals, e.g. squirrels, racoons, mice (Walton and Walls, 1964). Robertson's case was a woman of 29 who had one successful pregnancy in 1954 and abortions in 1959, 1960 and each of the two years after, producing a premature infant in 1961. Brain and placenta of the final foetus (twenty weeks) were inoculated into three mice, which all sickened and died of acute toxoplasmosis on the eighth day. Mice inoculated with this exudate died on the fourth day. The parasite was thus virulent. Robertson discusses the possible explanations of virulent parasites being isolated from a foetus of a mother with low or no antibody, and with a history of previous abortion. The main possibilities are:

1. Chronic toxoplasmosis in the mother with very low antibody titre.
2. Very recently acquired toxoplasmosis in the mother and previous abortions due to another cause.
3. Chronic toxoplasmosis and inability to form antibody—such as in a-gamma-globulinaemia.

4. Non-antigenicity of the strain.
5. Immune tolerance (Burnet, 1951, 1962).

But Beverley's findings (1959) suggest that there is no suppression of antibody in *T. gondii* in congenital infection of mice, even where the maternal infection was congenital. In Robertson's case, clearly, with no maternal antibody the infant would have no 'carry-over' antibody, and the parasites would not be sensitised before inoculation into the mice which succumbed so quickly—a point not made in the *Toxoplasma* literature but held to be of great importance in the production of virulent forms of *Treponema pallidum* by constant inoculation of parasites extracted from intra-testicular lesions less than ten days from inoculation, ten days being the time at which a new host produces effective antibody.

Previous isolations of *T. gondii* from foetuses, placentas, maternal tissues and fluids fall into three categories:

1. A brain-damaged infant shows perhaps histological evidence of toxoplasmosis, and maternal antibody titres are held to confirm this. Further, a history of maternal illness during the pregnancy has been assumed to be acute onset of toxoplasmosis in the mother. Subsequent pregnancies and births are normal (Sabin, 1949, 1952; Wright, 1957).
2. Isolation of *T. gondii* from foetuses and maternal tissues in cases of chronic abortion (Langer, 1963; Remington *et al.*, 1964; Wildfuhr, 1954, 1957; animals).
3. Accidental findings of the parasite in maternal tissues. Mellgren *et al.* (1952) saw *Toxoplasma*-like bodies in the routine histological examination of placentas in an investigation of neo-natal mortality, and confirmed that the maternal serum was *Toxoplasma*-inhibitory. The woman's history included a spontaneous abortion at 5/12, a premature infant, and a full-term child with a myelocoele. The final pregnancy ended in foetal death and an abnormal placenta, which they describe.

Langer's (1963) investigation of seventy women who had abortions or still-births yielded twenty-three with isolation of parasites, but only nineteen of these women had a positive dye-test. Two successive foetal brains from one mother yielded the parasite. The earliest pregnancies to abort were fourteen weeks; Langer does not state the foetal ages from the other women. Wernher *et al.* (1963) found histological evidence of parasites in the placenta at earlier dates (second and third months' abortions).

Remington *et al.* (1964) describe a patient who aborted an ovisac 1 × 3 cm, from whose curettings *T. gondii* was demonstrated, by inoculation into mice. The woman had a stable dye-test of 1/256—lower than those usually associated with acute toxoplasmosis. In 155 women (seventy-nine seronegative, thirty-four seropositive out of 113 tested), abortions, placentas, etc., were inoculated into mice, three yielding positive results.

Robertson's case does not differ greatly from these, except in the rapidity of effect on the mice and the absent dye-test titre. It is known that cases of retinal toxoplasmosis, from which parasites have been obtained, may be accompanied by low or even negative dye tests (Engelbrecht and Franceschetti, 1963).

It is reasonable to assume that, once encysted, antigenicity may fall, but if parasites are encysted—e.g. in the uterus, where tissue changes and stresses occur—rupture of the cyst might follow, yielding proliferative forms in a free field, uninhibited by antibody.

Immune response by the foetus It has been suggested by Burnet (1959, 1962) that, at a stage of foetal life, an immune tolerance might be established by the introduction of a foreign antigen.

In the human, evidence accrues of the ability to make certain antibody before birth: IgG may be 'maternal carry-over' but IgM is not, and is accepted as evidence of response to introduction of foreign antigen. Miller *et al.* (1967) have described their findings in two pairs of twins, one of each pair being severely affected by toxoplasmosis, the other relatively healthy though with a high dye-test titre. IgM was found as well as IgG in one of the diseased twins, but, in the healthy, IgG only. This could mean that the parasite only entered the diseased twin, establishing a foothold and calling forth some immune response, while the healthy twins had maternal antibody only.

The placenta as a barrier Gunders (1957) concluded that the extreme rarity of transplacental infection in man and animals made clear the efficiency of the placenta and foetal defences. In particular he was unable to transmit *T. gondii* RB strain during the last week of gestation to the foetuses, or RH strain during the last two days before littering, in mice and in rats. Beverley (1959) reported transmission to mice of the fourth and fifth generations.

Remington (1961) was able to record congenital transmission in chronically infected Sprague–Dawley rats to their young, none for RH or S6 strains, but RB strains transmitted one in ten, eight and six litter mates, two, four and eight months after infection. Mice gave occasional positive results for all strains. Guinea-pigs all produced negative foetuses. The author concluded that the guinea-pig placenta was not impermeable at any stage; and occasional infected foetuses were obtained from 'chronic' infections, where the guinea-pigs had been inoculated some months previously and the dye test was falling.

Transmission of the parasite in man
1. Congenital.
2. Acquired. The following suggestions have been made:
    (*a*) Raw meat eating (herbivorous animals could be infected from contaminated pastures). Against this is the fact that vegetarians acquire infection.
    (*b*) Insect vector, e.g. *Anopheles maculipennis* (Robertson, 1960). But Chapman (1967), although able to demonstrate that the mosquito took up the parasites, failed to demonstrate experimental infection from 'infected' bites.
    (*c*) Human secretions and excretions. *T. gondii* has been found in menstrual fluid, saliva (Cathie, 1954) and conjunctival secretions.
    (*d*) Droplet infection was suggested by Lainson (1955b) because of the presence of cysts in rabbit alveoli, and earlier reports by Pinkerton and Henderson (1941) in man.
    (*e*) Association with helminths (Hutchinson, 1965). Some significant increase in infection is achieved in cats with *Toxocara catis* ova: Woodruff (1968) points out other examples exist of helminths as vehicles and synergists of microbial infections.

Diagnosis of the infection
Diagnosis may be histological in lymphadenopathy (Stansfeld, 1961), but ideally isolation of parasite and confirmation of raised

dye-test titre would be required in all types of infection.

Isolation of the parasite, which is rarely recognisable in a human lesion, and rarely seen in its encysted form, is possible in mice. CSF or ground up and emulsified suspect tissue (in normal saline) is inoculated intraperitoneally in mice. These should be killed at three to four weeks and the brains examined for cysts. If a mouse dies earlier, peritoneal exudate and brain may be examined for proliferative forms, but a further inoculation from both should be done.

Two main serological tests are used to detect antibodies to *T. gondii*. The dye test of Sabin and Feldman (1948) consists of exposing *Toxoplasma* suspensions to methylene blue in the presence of the test serum, complement at 37°c and at pH 11. A non-immune patient's serum does not affect the normal uptake of dye; the serum of a patient who has the infection modifies the ability of the parasite to take up the dye. This antibody titre begins to rise ten to twenty days after infection. Complement fixation tests do not become positive till much later, never during acute illness.

Moyle (1967) has shown that the temperature at which the dye test is performed is critical: this may explain discrepancies between the results of different laboratories on the same sera.

Toxoplasmosis and deafness

Toxoplasmosis has not frequently been associated with deafness, nor with the pathology of the middle ear, the cochlea or the eighth nerve. Callahan, Russell and Smith (1946) described five fatal cases of congenital toxoplasmosis in young infants. Their case 2, a boy who died at the age of twelve weeks, was diagnosed at post-mortem as a case typical of toxoplasmosis encephalitis, with internal hydrocephalus and bilateral otitis media. During life he had initially presented the clinical syndrome of icterus gravis neonatorum: at the age of six weeks he began to cry continuously and developed ptosis of one eye, and convulsions. One tympanic membrane was slightly red and bulged. The cerebrospinal fluid was xanthochromic, with slightly increased protein and eighteen lymphocytes per cubic millimetre. By the age of nine weeks he had acute bilateral mastoiditis, for which he was operated on. During the next three weeks he deteriorated, vomiting copiously, and latterly was blind.

Sections of brain revealed extensive lesions with deformations of
the normal cortical architecture of the left cerebral hemisphere.
Large, vacuolated gitter cells, plasma cells and lymphocytes
packed the grey matter and were found less frequently in the
white. Several focal granulomatous areas were found, and toxoplasmata in and around these, in 'cysts' and singly. Calcification was
present in these areas. The Virchow–Robin space and the subarachnoid space were packed with lymphocytes and plasma cells. Sections
of the middle ears 'and a large part of the temporal bone' showed
very vascular granulation tissue in the operation wound, infiltrated
with polymorphonuclear leucocytes. There was marked destruction
of the bony trabeculae of the remaining left mastoid bone. Similar
changes were present on the right side. Toxoplasmata were identified in tissue from the left side, both within and outside cells. There
is no description of the cochlea nor of the condition of the eighth
nerve.

Cambell and Clifton (1950) described a rather unusual family,
when studying relatives of persons with serological or clinical
evidence of the disease. In three generations four persons suffered
from headache, periodic maculo-papular rash and nerve deafness.
Choroidoretinitis was present in affected members of the family.
Toxoplasma dye tests were positive in eight members of this family,
including those clinically affected, who also presented with 'saddle-
noses'. In view of the cough and joint pains, it seems likely that
some aetiology other than their toxoplasmosis was involved. The
Wassermann reaction of the cases was persistently negative. It is not
clear if this was on serum only, or on CSF. The CSF had raised
protein, raised pressure, and increased white cell counts. The authors
comment that in this family their choroidoretinitis was much more
slight and peripheral than that seen in some cases of toxoplasmosis,
where there is a large area affected near the macula. No improve-
ment in the headaches or rash or other symptoms was reported after
treatment. The dye-test titres were not very high, being 1/32 in two
cases and 1/128 in one. Brennan *et al.* (1949) described a rather
similar case, without nerve deafness, but commented on its similarity to periarteritis nodosa and erythema multiforme. It is also
possible that optic atrophy was secondary to papilloedema: further,
other causes of retinal degeneration and nerve deafness exist, and
they have not been excluded. It is now generally recognised that the

presence of antibody to *T. gondii* is widespread in human populations, with consequent positive dye tests.

Frenkel and Friedlander (1951) describe, in their case 7, otitis media and a wandering type of nystagmus, as well as chronic pharyngitis. Koch, Schorn and Ule (1951) describe bilateral mucous-suppurative otitis media in a child dying at three weeks, with intracranial calcifications, presumed to be toxoplasmic.

Dietzel (1958) examined deaf children with positive dye tests, and concluded that only in the presence of other clinical signs of toxoplasmosis could findings be significant.

Kelemen (1958) described two cases, one a premature infant dying at four weeks after birth, the other still-born. Both were considered as congenital toxoplasmosis, the maternal dye-test titres being 1/64, the second mother having had a maculopapular rash at 7/12 of pregnancy. In case 1, granulomatous lesions were found in the hydrocephalic brain, but organisms were not identified. In the middle ear, 'pseudocysts' and rosettes of parasites are mentioned. There were also deposits of calcium in the striae vascularis, which Kelemen considered reminiscent of the typical calcification of the cerebral hemispheres. The bone and sensory end-organs were, however, normal and mature for the developmental age. This case presented as hydrocephalic at two weeks, dying two weeks later. The maternal blood CFT was 1/64 (dye test not stated). The organisms were recovered from CSF. 'No infection or other gross pathology was present in the left middle ear' but the right petrous temporal bone was sectioned in toto: it revealed:

1. A deeply retracted but intact tympanic membrane.
2. Osseous walls of middle and internal ears were adequately developed for age, and sensory end organs normal.
3. Epitympanum filled with mesenchyme and transudate in which the three ossicles were embedded. The mucous membrane lining the tympanic cavity showed considerable thickening and in places cellular infiltration, but no engorgement and no extravasation. There were, however, 'rearrangement' buds. There was cellular infiltration round vessels, but also in avascular areas. A row of pseudocysts was found. Fibrous organisation was seen surrounding the incudomalleal joint 'like a plaster cast'.

4. In the internal ear a transudate was present, and mesenchymal remnants were identified in the semi-circular canals, though the cochlear canals were not affected thus, but Reissner's membrane was thought to be 'slightly depressed'.

5. The ganglionic areas of the canal of Rosenthal were empty in the areas corresponding to the upper half of the middle turn and the lower half of the apical.

6. Calcification of the stria vascularis was found in the middle turn and in the basal turn.

The second case, a 7/12 foetus, is in some ways similar in that an acute intra-uterine otitis media was present, in an infant with hydrocephalus. The mother had developed a maculopapular rash in the seventh month, which was treated with tetracycline and penicillin. No serological state in the mother is described.

Koch, Schorn and Ule's case (1951) at three weeks had similar features. Again the parasite was not recognised or isolated.

Thus the well documented cases of middle-ear disease due to toxoplasmosis are confined to cases of severe, widespread, congenital disease in which a temporal bone has been sectioned, namely, Kelemen's case 1 and Callahan *et al.*'s case 2.

Feinmesser and Landau's (1961) case is unlikely to be due to toxoplasmosis. A 14 year old boy had a retinal scar characteristic of the disease, and developed deafness at 7 years of age, perceptive in kind. The dye-test titre was 1/64, which is diagnostic only of past infection. They suggest that the perceptive deafness was possibly due to congenital toxoplasmosis, by analogy with choroidoretinitis.

Granz (1967) refers to 124 patients whose dye-test titres were 1/1,000, whom he considered to have acquired toxoplasmosis. He mentions two cases as 'florid, with inner-ear damage' but gives no further details.

Kubiczkowa (1962) examined 154 deaf children in Ostromecko, using the intradermal test of Frenkel: forty-two of the forty-nine positive children also had a positive complement fixation test. No comparison was made with the normal population, and x rays to detect cerebral calcification were negative. Similar suggestions appear in the literature from time to time, presumably on the analogy of the ophthalmic disease of toxoplasmosis congenitally acquired.

Inoculation of *T. gondii* into the middle ear of the guinea pig produces an acute inflammatory response, which resolves at the end of three weeks, and the infection becomes generalised (Wright, unpublished). Evidence of cochlear damage was not found. Transplanted transmission produced infection foetuses, but no pathology of the bulla or cochlea. Chick otocyst inoculation resulted in parasite multiplication in sensory cells and nerve fibres (Wright and Bird, unpublished).

References

Beattie, C.P. (1964), 'Toxoplasmosis', Lister Fellowship lecture, Roy. Coll. Physns. of Edinburgh.

— (1967), chapter on toxoplasmosis in *Recent Advances in Medical Microbiology*, ed. A. P. Waterson, Churchill, London.

Beverley, J.K.A., Skipper, E., and Marshall, S.C. (1955), *Brit. Med. Jl. 1*, 577.

Beverley, J.K.A. (1956), cited by Beattie (1957), *Trans. Roy. Soc. Trop. Med. Hyg. 51*, 57, 96.

— (1959), *Nature*, Lond. *183*, 1348.

Brennan, A.J., Brown, T., Warner, J., and Vrainien, E. (1949), *Amer. J. Med. 7*, 431.

Burnet, F.M. (1959), *Clonal Selection Theory of Acquired Immunity*, Cambridge University Press, London.

— (1962), *Brit. Med. Jl. 2*, 807.

Callahan, W.P., Russell, W.O., and Smith, M.G. (1946), *Medicine* (Baltimore), *25*, 343.

Campbell, A.M.C., and Clifton, F. (1950), *Brain, 73*, 281.

Castellani, A. (1914), *J. Trop. Med. 17*, 113.

Cathie, J.A. (1954), *Lancet, 2*, 115.

Chander, K., Mair, H.J., and Mair, N.S. (1968), *Brit. Med. Jl. 1*, 158.

Chapman, M. (1967), M. Phil. thesis, University of London.

Cook, M.K., and Jacobs, L. (1958), *J. Parasitol. 44*, 172.

Dietzel, K. (1958), *Arch. Ohr. Nas. Kehlk. 171*, 297.

Engelbrecht, E., and Franceschetti, A. (1963), *Path. et Microbiol. 26*, 731.

Feinmesser, M., and Landau, J. (1961), *J. Laryng. 75*, 171.

Frenkel, J.K., and Friedlander, S. (1951), *Publ. Hlth. Serv. publication No. 141*, N.I.H., Washington, D.C.

Fulton, J.D. (1967), *Lab. Animals, 1*, 7.

Granz, W. (1967), *Münsch. Med. Wschr. 109*, 715.

Gunders, A.E.L. (1957), Ph.D. thesis, University of London.
Hogan, M.J., Zweigart, P., and Lewis, A. (1958), *Arch. Ophthal. 60*, 548.
Hutchinson, W.M. (1965), *Nature*, Lond. *206*, 961.
Kelemen, G. (1958), *Arch. Otolaryng. 68*, 547.
Kirchoff, H. (ed.) (1967), *Toxoplasmose Symposium, Gottingen*, Thieme, Stuttgart.
Koch, F., Schorn, J., and Ule, G. (1951), *Deutsch. Z. Nervenh. 166*, 316.
Kubiczkowa, J. (1962), *Otolaryng. Polsk. 16*, 4.
Lainson, R. (1955a), *Ann. Trop. Med. Parasitol. 49*, 397.
— (1955b), *Trans. Roy. Soc. Trop. Med. Hyg. 49*, 296.
— (1959), *Ann. Trop. Med. Parasit. 53*, 120.
Langer, H. (1963), *Am. J. Obst. Gynec. 21*, 318.
Mellgren, J., Alm, L., and Kjessler, A. (1952), *Acta Path. Microb. Scand. 30*, 59.
Miller, M.J., Seaman, E., and Remington, J.S. (1967), *Pediatrics, 70*, 714.
Moyle, G.G. (1967), *Aust. J. Exp. Biol. Med. Sci. 45*, 571.
Nicolle, C., and Manceaux, L. (1908), *C. R. Acad. Sci. 147*, 763; *148*, 369.
Pinkerton, H., and Henderson, R. (1941), *J. Amer. M. H. 116*, 807.
Rawal, B.D. (1959), *J. Clin. Path. 12*, 59.
Remington, J.S., Melton, M.L., and Jacobs, L. (1960), *J. Lab. Clin. Med. 56*, 879.
— (1961), *J. Immunol. 87*, 578.
Remington, J.S. (1961) in toxoplasmosis symposium, *Survey Ophthal.* 6, ed. Maumenee, A.E.
Remington, J.S., Newell, J.W., and Cavanagh, E. (1964), *Obst. Gynec. 24*, 25.
Robertson, J.S. (1960), *Brit. Med. Jl. 2*, 91.
— (1962), *Develop. Med. Child Neurol. 4*, 507.
— (1965), *J. Hyg. Camb. 63*, 89.
— (1966), *Postgrad. Med. Jl. 42*, 61.
Rowland, L.P., and Greer, M. (1961), *Neurology* (Minneapolis), *11*, 367.
Sabin, A.B., and Feldman, H.A. (1948), *Science, 108*, 660.
Sabin, A.B. (1949), *Pediatrics, 4*, 443.
— (1950), *Trans. Amer. Acad. Ophth. Otolaryng. 54*, 190.
Sabin, A.B., Eichenwald, H., Feldman, H.A., and Jacobs, L. (1952), *Jl. Amer. Med. Assn. 150*, 1053.

Sexton, R.C., Eyles, D.E., and Dillman, R.E. (1953), *Amer. J. Med. 14*, 366.

Sheffield, H.G., and Melton, M.L. (1968), *J. Parasitol. 54*, 209.

Siim, J. (1961), *Survey Ophthal. 6*, 781.

Stansfeld, A.G. (1961), *J. Clin. Path. 14*, 573.

Vischer, T.L., Bernheim, C., and Engelbrecht, E. (1967), *Lancet, 2*, 919.

Walton, B.C., and Walls, K.W. (1964), *Am. J. Trop. Med. Hyg. 13*, 530.

Werner, H. (1962), *Z. Zbl. Bakt. Orig. 186*, 391.

Werner, H., Schmidtke, L., and Thomaschek, G. (1963), *Klin. Wschr. 41*, 96.

Wildfuhr, G. (1954), *Z. Immunitätforsch, 111*, 110.

— (1957), *Toxoplasmose*, Fischer, Stuttgart.

Woodruff, A.W. (1968), *Trans. Roy. Soc. Trop. Med. Hyg. 62*, 446.

Wright, I., and Bird, E.S. (unpublished).

Wright, W.H. (1957), *Am. J. Clin. Path. 28*, 1.

XX Diseases of the reticulo-endothelial system

Leukaemia, Waldenstrom's macroglobulinaemia and other disorders of these systems may produce defects of hearing by:

1. Lowered immunity and susceptibility to infection.
2. Thrombocytopaenia (due to invasion of the bone marrow by neoplastic cells), which may encourage bleeding into the cochlea.

Macroglobulinaemia may affect the cochlea by both these mechanisms, and possibly may affect the fluid in the cochlear canals by the presence of abnormal protein. Ronis *et al.* (1966) describe two clinical cases with cochlear and vestibular involvement. They suggest stagnation of blood flow, haemorrhage, and thrombosis of the vessels. They refer to other cases where labyrinthine involvement appeared to be a presenting feature. Logothetis *et al.* (1960) found seven cases with hearing loss in 182 cases with neurologic manifestations.

References

Logothetis, J., Silverstein, P., and Coe, J. (1960), *Arch. Neurol. 3*, 564.
Ronis, M.L., Rojer, C.L., and Ronis, B.J. (1966), *Laryngoscope, 76*, 513.

XXI Brief biographies and a few historical notes on the investigation of hearing

Much of the early work on the inner ear, e.g. Kerkringius (1670), is described by Bast and Anson in *The Temporal Bone and the Ear*.

Leonardo da Vinci, 1452–1519

During the first phase of his career in Milan as an anatomist Leonardo developed his knowledge of the cranial nerves. He was aware of the cerebral ventricles, the optic chiasma and the eyeballs. Primarily interested in nerves and muscles and eyes as a means of expression of the mind, he was aware of some of the cranial nerves, e.g. branches of the maxillary division of the trigeminal nerve (f. B35).

Later, in Florence, he points out that the function of the optic nerves is known to him: they carry what the eye perceives to the *senso communo*. He argued from this that the soul is confined to the *senso communo* and not, as previously believed, in the whole body, or there could be no need for optic nerves as the eyes would enable the soul to perceive and comprehend on the surface of the eye. He makes similar comments on the senses of hearing and smell (f. B2r).

Although his drawings show his careful dissections of some of the cranial nerves, and particularly the end-organ of sight, he was apparently unaware of the seventh cranial nerve and probably the eighth: he has left no dissection of the temporal bone (f. B).

In fact Leonardo da Vinci seems to have known little more than Galen on hearing. The cavity of complicated form within the petrous temporal bone was necessary for the resounding of a voice if it were to be heard. There is no suggestion that he explored the labyrinth, but he associated a pair of nerves with carrying sound to the *sensus communis*. (K. D. Keele in *Essays on the History of Italian Neurology*, ed. Belloni, the Proceedings of the Int. Symp.

Hist. of Neurology (1961) at Varenna, Milan, 1963. 'Dell'anatomia, fogli B', *I manoscritti di Leonardo da Vinci della Reale Biblioteca di Windsor*; an edition published in Milan in 1901 by T. Sabachnikov exists.)

Alfonso Corti, 1822–76

Salvatore Iurato, in a paper entitled 'The neurological work of Alfonso Corti' (*Symposium on the History of Italian Neurology*, Varenna, 1961), states that Corti used the freshest possible material from the still warm animal. He placed the tissue between two slides, bonded with a mastic following Harting's method. Fixative was then run in, sometimes followed by carmine. Iurato says that Corti was the first to use carmine as a histological stain. The magnifications he was able to use were from 20 × to 500 ×.

In 1845 Todd and Bowman, and in the same year Huschke, had published cursory and confused references to the stria vascularis, sensory epithelium and the tectorial membrane.

In 1851 Corti published 'Recherches sur l'organe de l'ouie des mammifères' in *Zeitschr. f. wissen. Zool. 3*, 109–209.

He was the first to describe the stria vascularis, and to suggest that the capillaries sheathed with epithelial cells, of which the stria is formed, were responsible for the endolymph.

He appears to have missed the inner hair-cells in some preparations but noted that the apical outer hair-cells were longest, and the basal shortest. It is this work which justifies the use of Corti's name in the anatomical title of the spiral end-organ of hearing.

He entered medical school at Pavia, and four years later went to Hyrtl's department of anatomy at Vienna, producing a doctoral thesis in 1847. Hyrtl's advice led him later to investigate the inner ear.

In 1848, of course, it was expedient to move, and he went to Zurich. He continued his work on the ear and started on the retina, on which he published a paper in 1850. He resumed his work on the ear in Kolliker's department at Wurtzburg, and later to Harting's Observatorium at Utrecht. With the methods acquired there he returned to Wurtzburg and Paris and completed his work on the ear (1851). He went to Turin, to the Zoological Laboratory, and communicated his results to Kölliker, who published them, with comments, in 1854.

He married in 1855 and retired to Mezzolino, where he lived until 1876. His only publications were:

1850. 'Anatomie des retina', *Archiv. fur. Anat. Physiol. u. wissen Medizin.*

1851. The paper (*q.v. supra*) on the mammalian organ of hearing.

1852. Kölliker used his drawing of a bipolar cell of the spiral ganglion in *Historie der Gewebelehre des Menschen*, Leipzig, Engelmann (Fig. 311 in that work).

1854. *Ztsch. f. wiss. Zool.* 5, 87–93, a joint paper, with Prof. A. Kölliker, on sensory nerve cells in the elephant.

Gustav Magnus Retzius, 1842–1919

'Did more to enrich anatomical literature than any other man of his time' (Sir Arthur Keith, in the obituary published in *Nature*, vol. 103, p. 448, 1919). His grandfather had been professor of anatomy at Lund, his father, Anders Retzius, at the Karolinska Institute, Stockholm. It is to Anders Retzius that we owe the classification of human skull types by the ratio of breadth to length. Gustav Retzius was, like his father, an ethnologist and anthropologist as well as an anatomist.

He published *Das Gehörorgan der Wirbelthieren* (Stockholm, 1881–84) after many years' work. In volume II, describing the hearing organs of reptiles, birds and mammals, there are plates which include the surface views of the spiral organ which we associate with his name. The description of the human organ begins on p. 328; the plates are XXXIII–XXXIX. Tables recording sizes of cells and lengths of various parts of the spiral organ and the membranous cochlea are found on pp. 354–56.

Joseph Toynbee, 1815–66

The son of a Lincolnshire farmer, he was a nineteenth century aural surgeon with a keen interest in aetiology and the pathology of aural disease. His collection of temporal bones was lost in the second world war. He was a keen observer of all forms of natural history, and encouraged its study by others, founding a museum at Wimbledon, where he himself lectured weekly to the forerunners of the adult education movement. He was a supporter of the Bedford Institutes, which continue the educational work of Peter Bedford. (Toynbee Hall, which was founded in 1884, with similar aims, was, however, named to commemorate Arnold Toynbee, the social philosopher and economic historian, who was Joseph Toynbee's second son, and died at about thirty years of age in 1883 (see Pinlott).)

Joseph Toynbee, who was apprenticed to William Wade, a surgeon in Gerrard Street, Soho, became a member of the Royal College of Surgeons in 1838. He worked at St George's Hospital and University College. His work on the non-vascular tissues earned his Fellowship of the Royal Society in 1842: it is to be found in the *Philosophical Transactions* of 1841.

He was for many years on the staff of St Mary's Hospital, but after a disagreement with the governors was appointed to the Midland Ear and Throat Hospital at Birmingham in 1862. Four years later he died of chloroform overdose and possibly hydrocyanic acid, experimenting with these substances in a search for an alleviation of tinnitus (Stevenson and Guthrie). (See also Guthrie's presidential address, 1936, Simpson's, 1962, and Cawthorne's commemoration of Toynbee at the Section of Otology meeting at Edinburgh in 1966, reported in volume 80 of the *Journal of Laryngology and Otology*.)

Temporal bone sections

It seems probable that Politzer was the first to cut temporal bone sections as we know them today. In 1881 Steinbrügge published an illustration of parts of the labyrinth seen at different levels, but the 'sections' are thick enough to have been cut by hand, with a saw.

By 1903 Alexander produced good mid-modiolar sections cut at 15–20 microns from a celloidin-embedded temporal bone (see also Alexander, 1896). In 1925 Alexander and Fischer pay tribute to Politzer's 1889 publication as a great step forward in the microscopical examination of the human ear.

It appears likely that J. S. Fraser of Edinburgh introduced temporal bone sectioning into the United Kingdom.

References

Alexander, G. (1896), *Z. J. Wissensch. Mikros. M. Tek.*, XIII.
— (1903), *Z. Ohrenheilk. 61*, 185.
Alexander, G., and Fischer, J. (1925), *Präparationstechnik des Gehör-organes mit Berücksichtingung des Nachbargebietes*, Urban and Schwarzenberg.
Bast, C.H., and Anson, B.J. (1949), *The Temporal Bone and the Ear*, Thomas, Springfield, Ill.
Gardner's Pathology of Connective Tissue Diseases. Thomas, Springfield, Ill.
Major, R.H., *Classic Descriptions of Disease*, Thomas, Springfield, Ill.
Pinlott, J.A.R. (1935), *Toynbee Hall: Fifty Years of Progress*, Dent, London.
Politzer, A. (1889), *Uber die anatomische und histologische Zergliede-rung des Menschlichen Ohres*, Enke, Stuttgart.
Steinbrugge, H. (1881), *Z. Ohrenheilk*, plate v.
Stevenson, R.S., and Guthrie, D.J. (1949), *History of Otolaryngology*, Livingstone, Edinburgh.

A low viscosity nitrocellulose method for cutting sections of the temporal bone

Fixation. Fix for three weeks in formol saline.

Wash overnight

Decalcification. Decalcify in the following solution for six to eight weeks, controlling by x-ray towards the end of this period:

Formic acid 98 per cent	368 ml.
Sodium formate	86 g.
Tap water to	2000 ml.

Fluid should be changed every two to three days at first and then weekly.

Neutralisation. Transfer to 5 per cent sodium sulphate for twenty-four hours. Wash in running water forty-eight hours.

Dehydration. Dehydrate as follows:

70 per cent alcohol	24 hours
90 per cent alcohol	24 hours
96 per cent alcohol	72 hours (× 3 changes)
Absolute alcohol I	24 hours
Absolute alcohol II	24 hours
Absolute alcohol III	24 hours
Fresh alcohol	24 hours
Absolute alcohol and ether 50/50	48 hours

Impregnation.	5 per cent low viscosity nitrocellulose	21 days
	10 per cent low viscosity nitrocellulose	14 days
	20 per cent low viscosity nitrocellulose	14 days

Embedding. Place specimen in square museum jar with flat surface downwards. Pour over it sufficient 20 per cent low viscosity nitrocellulose plus 1 per cent dibutyl phthalate to cover and leave half an inch or so around the specimen. Treat the ground glass lid with Vaseline and place on jar. Allow LVN to solidify slowly by raising the lid for a short period each day, until a skin has formed on the surface. Treat with chloroform vapour until a hard surface has formed. Add more chloroform and leave until the block has become solid right through. Allow the block to shrink by draining off the chloroform and allowing it to dry. Remove from jar and store in 70 per cent alcohol for at least three to four days before cutting.

Mounting of block on holder. Soften base of LVN block in 20 per cent LVN by constant agitation for at least ten minutes. Pour 20 per cent LVN over Stabilite block and place the LVN block in position, keeping the pressure on with the aid of a 500 gram weight until the outer surface is dry.

    Place in 70 per cent alcohol overnight with the weight still in position.

Cutting. Sections can be cut at about 20 microns or less on a sledge-type microtome. They are removed from the knife and placed into 70 per cent alcohol. Every tenth section is stained.

Staining

1. Stain in Ehrlich's haematoxylin—75 minutes to 3 hours.
2. Blue in 'tap water substitute'—20 minutes.
3. Differentiate in 1 per cent acid alcohol—10 seconds.
4. Blue in 'tap water substitute'.
5. Stain in 0·05 per cent eosin—20 minutes.
6. Wash briefly in tap water.
7. Treat with 70 per cent alcohol.
8. Pick up on slide.
9. Treat with 96 per cent alcohol.
10. Treat with fresh 96 per cent alcohol. Blot.
11. Treat with Carbol–Xylol. (Phenol, 25 g; Xylol, 75 ml.) Blot.
12. Treat with Xylol.
13. Mount in Xam.

Note. Sections may be stored in 70 per cent alcohol.

Serial sections are numbered by using a lead pencil on special Vellin tissue (obtainable from General Paper & Box Manufacturing Co. Ltd, Pontypridd, Glam.).

References

Kristensen, H.K. (July 1948), *Stain Technology*, *23*, 151.

Chesterman, W., and Leach, E.H. (1949), *Quart. J. Micro. Sci.* 90, 431.

Chesterman, W., and Leach, E.H. (1950), *Quart. J. Med. Sci.*

Chesterman, W. (October 1950), *Bull. Inst. Med. Lab. Tech.* *15*, 5, 88.

Index